Quick Reference Dictionary
of
Eyecare Terminology

THIRD EDITION

Joseph Hoffman

Janice K. Ledford, COMT

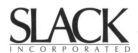

An innovative information, education and management company
6900 Grove Road • Thorofare, NJ 08086

Library of Congress Cataloging-in-Publication Data

Hoffman, Joseph,
  Quick reference glossary of eyecare terminology / Joseph Hoffman,
  Janice K. Ledford.--3rd ed.
    p. ; cm.
  Includes bibliographical references.
    ISBN 1-55642-472-8 (alk. paper)
    1. Ophthalmology--Dictionaries.
    [DNLM: 1. Eye Diseases--therapy--Terminology--English. 2.
  Ophthalmology--Terminology--English. WW 15 H699q 2002] I. Ledford,
  Janice K. II. Title.
  RE21 .H64 2002
  617.7'003--dc21
                                          2002008822

0027892

Printed in the United States of America.
Published by: SLACK Incorporated
                     6900 Grove Road
                     Thorofare, NJ 08086 USA
                     Telephone: 856-848-1000
                     Fax: 856-853-5991
                     www.slackbooks.com

  Contact SLACK Incorporated for more information about other books in this field or about the availability of our books from distributors outside the United States.

  For permission to reprint material in another publication, contact SLACK Incorporated. Authorization to photocopy items for internal, personal, or academic use is granted by SLACK Incorporated provided that the appropriate fee is paid directly to Copyright Clearance Center. Prior to photocopying items, please contact the Copyright Clearance Center at 222 Rosewood Drive, Danvers, MA 01923 USA; phone: 978-750-8400; website: www.copyright.com; email: info@copyright.com

  Last digit is print number: 10 9 8 7 6 5 4 3 2 1

DEDICATION

Dedicated, for my part, to the Mighty Girl Writers:
Londa, Pam, Eva, and Dee.
Jan Ledford

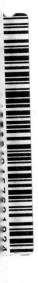

CONTENTS

Dedication . . . . *v*
Acknowledgments . . . . *ix*
About the Authors. . . . . *xi*
Preface. . . . . *xiii*

Dictionary of Terms 1

Appendix 1:	Acronyms and Abbreviations . 195
Appendix 2:	Medical Terminology 209
Appendix 3:	The Schematic Eye 215
Appendix 4:	The Cranial Nerves 217
Appendix 5:	Classifications of Nystagmus . . 219
Appendix 6:	Red Eye Differential Diagnosis . 221
Appendix 7:	The Subjective Grading System 225
Appendix 8:	Slit Lamp Findings for Systemic Diseases and Conditions 233
Appendix 9:	Systemic Disorders and Their Effects On the Eye 239
Appendix 10:	Ophthalmic Drugs 247
Appendix 11:	Lasers in Ophthalmology 279
Appendix 12:	Ocular and Systemic Effects of Topical Ocular Drugs. 283
Appendix 13:	Normal Values of Common Blood Tests 287
Appendix 14:	The Metric System 289
Appendix 15:	English and Metric Conversion 293
Appendix 16:	Weights and Measures. 295
Appendix 17:	Manual Alphabet for Communicating With the Hearing Impaired. 297
Appendix 18:	The Braille Alphabet 299

Appendix 19:   Certification as Paraoptometric
                and Ophthalmic Medical
                Personnel. 301
Appendix 20:   Websites Related to Eyecare . . 309
Appendix 21:   Suggested Reading. 321

ACKNOWLEDGMENTS

Taking on the third and subsequent editions of this book meant that I will forever build on the work of Joe Hoffman. I thank him for establishing the foundation. Thank you to SLACK Incorporated employees Amy McShane, Debra Toulson, and John Bond for handing me this project. Others who helped are Tiffany K. Spooner, Paraoptometric Section of the AOA, for providing updated information on paraoptometric assistants; Art Giebel, MD, Loma Linda University Medical Center, a contact of Joe's, for providing abbreviations; Bernie Calaway for proofreading assistance and general encouragement; Jim Ledford, my husband, who understands; and Collin Ledford, our teenaged son, who also understands and even does some writing of his own.

—*Jan Ledford, COMT*

ABOUT THE AUTHORS

Joseph Hoffman has worked in medical publishing since 1985 and was the editor-in-chief of the *Ocular Surgery News* publication group from 1996 to 2001. He has won writing awards from the American Society of Business Publication Editors and Apex. He is currently the proprietor of Hoffman Health Care Communications.

For over 20 years now, *Jan Ledford* has been using her skills both in the ophthalmic exam room and on the printed page. While she is probably best known for her certification review books and editorship of *The Basic Bookshelf for Eyecare Professionals*, she is also a published novelist. She recently combined her talent for medical research with that of story telling to produce *The Cloning*, a novel about human cloning, which is available at book stores everywhere as well as online. In spite of branching out, she has no intentions of leaving the field of eyecare, where, she says, she has found a permanent and happy home.

PREFACE

I am way past grammar school, believe me, but the words "Go look it up" still strike terror in my heart. Not because I do not *like* to look up new terms—far from it. The problem is that I cannot look up just *one*! I get side-tracked right away with interesting-looking entries that I just might want to use someday. In the interest of expediency, it is much easier to have someone *tell* me the meaning.

Medicine has its own unique breed of terms, founded from Greek, Latin, and who knows where else. The current *Stedman's Medical Dictionary* is a two-volume set... a place where I could easily get lost and spend many happy hours, if I just had the time.

Many of you in eyecare share my delight; others do not. Here is a single volume containing all things optic (well, lots anyway) plus a smattering of general medical terms to get you by. If you are new to the field, there's a lot to learn. If you're an old-timer (might we coin a new term here: presbytech?), there is something new right around every optic, ophthalmic, and optometric corner.

The task of taking on SLACK Incorporated's ophthalmic dictionary, like most projects, turned out to be bigger than I thought. Not the least of these is a simple difference of opinion on some of the words themselves: Is it Grave disease, Graves disease, or Grave's disease? I found references that confirmed each and every one, and doubtless some of you won't agree with the spelling I selected. Then there are your personal pet obscure terms that I left in (spiral of Tillaux is one of mine, so it got in) and obsolete words that made the cut (such as squint). Others might argue that the inclusion of some general medical terms takes the book needlessly beyond the realm of eyecare.

In the final analysis, all I can offer is one of my favorite (and original) axioms regarding publishing: There is no such thing as a perfect book.

Regardless, a lot of people worked really hard to make this one come as close as possible. Meanwhile, I'm starting on the fourth edition, and I'd appreciate your input. Please email me at educomps@slackinc.com to share your ideas on what terms should be added and deleted, what new appendices would be most helpful, those definitions that need improvement, alternate spellings, typos—whatever! Together, we'll continue to make *The Quick Reference Dictionary of Eyecare Terminology* the most turned-to word reference book in the field.

—*Jan Ledford, COMT*
July 8, 2002

A-constant: 1. Number assigned to an intraocular lens (IOL) by the manufacturer based on the lens design; used in formulas for calculating power of IOL needed in a given patient; 2. number derived from actual visual results of IOL implantation by a particular surgeon; used as part of subsequent IOL power calculations to "personalize" the formula and better reflect the influence of surgeon technique.

"A" measurement: The horizontal eye size of a pair of spectacles, measured in millimeters from one side of the eyewire to the other; *see also* boxing system.

A pattern esotropia: *See* esotropia *and* exotropia.

A-scan: As used in ophthalmology, an ultrasound examination to determine the axial length of the eye (distance from the front of the cornea to the back of the retina) and possibly the depth of various intraocular structures; most commonly used in calculating the power of intraocular lenses.

ab externo: General medical term meaning *from the outside*; in ophthalmic usage, describing surgical procedures in which the approach to an anatomic structure is made from outside the globe.

Abbe value: A rating (from 1 to 100) that indicates the amount of chromatic aberration present in a lens material; a higher number indicates less likelihood of aberration; also called *Nu value.*

abducens nerve: Sixth cranial nerve; supplies the lateral rectus muscle.

abduct: General medical term for inducing motion away from the center of the body; in ophthalmic usage, muscles that move an eye toward the temple are called *abductors; compare* adduct.

aberration: Uneven refraction of light in an optical system resulting in distortion of the transmitted image; *see also* chromatic aberration *and* spherical aberration.

ablation: General medical term for destruction of tissue (usually as part of a surgical procedure); in laser surgery, vaporization of tissue by the laser.

abnormal retinal correspondence (ARC): *See* anomalous retinal correspondence.

abrasion: General medical term for wound in which layers of tissue are scraped away; in ophthalmic usage, often used as a synonym for corneal abrasion.

accommodation: Adjustment of focal power of the eye from distance to near vision achieved by contraction of the ciliary muscle, which causes a thickening of the crystalline lens and a slight forward shift in its position, both of which increase its refractive power; **absolute a.** accommodation of either eye independently; **binocular a.** uniform accommodation of both eyes together in convergence (ie, the inward turning of both eyes in viewing a near object); **convergence a.** accommodation that occurs in either eye upon convergence; **far point of a.** distance from the eye to the farthest point clearly visible when accommodation is relaxed; **near point of a.** distance from the eye to the nearest point clearly visible when accommodation is at its maximum; **negative a.** relaxation of accommodation for distance vision; **positive a.** exercise of accommodation for near vision; **range of a.** the distance between the near and far points of accommodation.

accommodative amplitude (AA): The amount of accommodation (measured in diopters) required at the near point of accommodation.

accommodative convergence (AC): Inward turning of both eyes that normally occurs in response to accommodation.

accommodative convergence/accommodation (AC/A): The relationship (a ratio) between the amount that the eyes turn inward (accommodative convergence, measured in prism diopters) and the increase in their focusing power (accommodation, measured in diopters) that occurs when viewing a near object, calculated as accommodative convergence divided by accommodation; *see also* accommodation *and* convergence.

accommodative insufficiency (AI): Abnormal weakening of the accommodation reflex; may be due to injury, disease, or the effects of medication.

accommodative miosis: Normal constriction of pupils associated with accommodation.

accommodative spasm: Accommodation without subsequent relaxation of the ciliary muscle, resulting in a prolonged state of near focus (rendering distant objects unclear).

acetylcholine: Biochemical (neurotransmitter) that activates the parasympathetic nervous system; in the eye, it stimulates the ciliary muscle and the sphincter muscle of the iris; *see also* cholinergic; *compare* epinephrine *and* norepinephrine.

achromatic lens: An ophthalmic lens that is free from chromatic aberration (ie, it does not break light into its component colors).

achromatism: A condition in which all three visual pigments are absent; also known as *rod monochromatism*; complete color blindness; *compare* dichromatism, monochromatism, *and* trichromatism.

acorea: Absence of the pupil.

acrylic: Of or relating to acrylic acid or its many derivative compounds; in eyecare, usually an optically clear polymer used in the manufacture of lenses.

acrylic lens implant: *See* intraocular lens.

acuity: Clarity of vision; specifically, the ability to distinguish fine details; often expressed as a score on Snellen's, Jaeger's, or other vision testing charts.

acute: In medical usage, denoting the immediate or severe; *compare* chronic; *see* entries under main word (eg, *see* glaucoma for acute angle-closure glaucoma, etc).

adaptation: General medical term for adjustment to changing conditions; specifically in ophthalmic usage: **color a.** adjustment of vision to bright colors such that the color intensity diminishes with time; **dark a.** adjustment of vision in dim light, primarily by increasing levels of rhodopsin (visual purple) in the rods of the retina, making the eye more sensitive to light; *see* scotopia; **light a.** adjustment of vision in bright light by decreasing levels of light-sensitive pigments of the retina; *see* photopia; **photopic a.** another term for light a.; **retinal a.** general term for adjustment of vision to varying light conditions; **scotopic a.** *see* dark a.

add: 1. Amount of additional refractive power needed in spectacles or contact lenses (prescribed for distance vision correction) to correct a presbyopic eye for near (ie, "reading") vision; 2. the portion of a lens that is designed to provide that additional near corrective power; *see also* segment.

adduct: General medical term for inducing motion toward the center of the body; in ophthalmic usage, muscles that move an eye toward the nose are called *adductors*; *compare* abduct.

Adie's pupil or **syndrome:** Uneven contraction of the pupils of each eye upon accommodation (in near vision) in which the affected pupil reacts poorly to light and slowly to near; also called *tonic pupil* or *myotonic pupil*.

adjustable suture: Suture placed in glaucoma, refractive, or other surgery to allow tightening or loosening in the postoperative period to modify the results of surgery.

adnexa: General anatomic term for the structures surrounding an organ; the ocular adnexa are usually considered to include the eyelids, lacrimal apparatus, orbits, and other tissues within the orbits.

adrenaline: Another term for epinephrine.

adrenergic: Substance or system that stimulates the sympathetic nervous system; also called *sympathomimetic*; phenylephrine (a mydriatic) is an adrenergic drug; *compare* cholinergic.

advancement: In ophthalmic usage, operation (usually for correction of strabismus) in which an extraocular muscle or tendon is detached and repositioned more anteriorly to increase its action; **capsular a.** surgical manipulation of Tenon's capsule in order to achieve advancement of an extraocular muscle.

afferent pupillary defect (APD): Another term for Marcus Gunn pupil.

after-cataract: *See* capsular opacification.

afterimage: Perception of an image that persists after the visual stimulus ends; **complementary a.** afterimage in which the persisting colors are complementary to the colors of the original visual stimulus; **negative a.** afterimage in which bright elements of a visual stimulus persist as dark and dark elements become light; **positive a.** afterimage in which light elements persist as light and dark elements remain dark.

against-the-rule astigmatism (ATR): *See* astigmatism.

age-related macular degeneration (ARMD or AMD): *See* macular degeneration.

agonist: The muscle receiving primary innervation to contract (eg, the lateral rectus in abduction); *compare* antagonist.

air-fluid exchange: *See* gas-fluid exchange.

air-puff tonometer: *See* tonometer.

akinesia: General term for lack of motion or inability to move; most often in ophthalmic usage, referring to the lack of voluntary movement of the eye following retrobulbar or peribulbar anesthesia.

alexia: The inability to understand written language; also called *word blindness*.

Allen cards, chart, or **test:** Visual acuity test employing pictures to assess the vision of young children and the mentally challenged.

allergic conjunctivitis: *See* conjunctivitis.

alpha angle: *See* angle.

alpha chymotrypsin: Enzyme injected into the anterior chamber to dissolve zonular fibers and facilitate intracapsular cataract extraction.

alternate cover test: *See* cover test.

alternating amblyopia: *See* amblyopia.

alternating strabismus: *See* strabismus.

amacrine cells: Nerve cells that are found in the inner nuclear layer of the retina; *see also* retina.

amaurosis: General term for blindness, usually referring to blindness caused by some defect apart from the tissues of the eyeball; **central a.** temporary blindness resulting from disease or defect of the central nervous system; **hysterical a.** temporary blindness resulting from neurosis; **sympathetic a.** blindness in one eye occurring because of disease in the other eye.

amaurosis fugax: A temporary state (about 10 minutes or so) of partial or full blindness in one eye often associated with carotid artery disease.

amaurotic nystagmus: Rapid involuntary movements of a blind eye.

amaurotic pupil: Pupil that does not respond to direct light stimulation but does dilate and constrict when the fellow eye receives light stimulus; an eye with an amaurotic pupil is blind, usually because of damage to the optic nerve or retina.

amblyope: One who suffers from amblyopia.

amblyopia: Impaired vision in one or both eyes that cannot be remedied with corrective lenses and has no obvious organic cause in the structures of the eye or visual pathway (colloquially known as *lazy eye*); **alcoholic a.** amblyopia caused by alcohol toxicity (also known as *amblyopia crapulosa*); **alternating a.** diminished vision occurring in the nonfixating eye in alternating strabismus; **ametropic a.** *see* refractive a.; **anisometropic a.** amblyopia arising from a significant difference in the refractive power of the two eyes in which the eye requiring the greatest accommodation to achieve clear vision becomes disused; **astigmatic a.** refractive amblyopia occurring because of uncorrected astigmatism; **color a.** general term for impairment of color vision; **crossed a.** amblyopia in one eye with loss of feeling in the opposite side of the face (also known as *amblyopia cruciata*); **deprivation a.** amblyopia following a period in which central fixation was lost due to cataract, drooping eyelid, etc (also known as *amblyopia of disuse*); called **occlusion a.** when central fixation was intentionally obstructed (as with an eye patch); **functional** or **reversible a.** amblyopia that can be corrected with eyeglasses or occlusion of the opposite eye in childhood; **nocturnal a.** *see* nyctalopia; **reflex a.** amblyopia resulting from some insult or injury to the eye; **refractive a.** due to a high uncorrected refractive error; also called *ametropic amblyopia*; **strabismic a.** amblyopia arising from strabismus in which one eye becomes preferred over the other, which then falls into disuse; **suppression a.** amblyopia resulting from deprivation of sight in an eye by ptosis, cataract, corneal opacity, etc; also called *amblyopia ex anopsia*, *deprivation amblyopia*, or *amblyopia of disuse*.

ametropia: General term for conditions in which the eye does not focus properly but can be corrected with eyeglasses or other vision aids, commonly called a *refractive error* (*see* astigmatism, hyperopia, myopia, *and* presbyopia); **axial a.** ametropia attributable to the length of the eyeball (too long in myopia or too short in hyperopia); **curvature a.** ametropia attributable to corneal curvature (too steep in myopia or too flat in hyperopia); **position a.** ametropia attributable to the position of the crystalline lens of the eye (too far forward in myopia or too far back in hyperopia); **refractive a.** general term for any ametropia attributable to an error in the eye's system for focusing light rays on the retina; *compare* emmetropia.

amplitude of accommodation: *See* accommodative amplitude.

amplitude of convergence: Maximum angle to which the eyes can turn inward (from parallel lines of sight in distance vision) toward the nose to fix upon a nearby object.

Amsler grid or **chart (AG):** Visual field testing grid consisting of evenly spaced horizontal and vertical lines, typically white lines on a dark background with a central dot to mark the point of fixation; used as a simple test for detecting defects or distortions in the central 20 degrees of the visual field.

amyloid body: Deposit of abnormal starch-protein compound seen in amyloidosis.

amyloidosis: Condition in which deposits of amyloid accumulate in various body tissues, including the vitreous humor and ocular nerves and blood vessels.

anaglyph: Vision test target consisting of two similar images with different portions printed in red, green, and sometimes black; subject views each image separately with each eye, and a red filter is placed before one eye and a green filter before the other; patient reports the image seen, providing a measure of fusion and stereoscopic function.

analgesic: Drug that relieves pain without rendering the patient unconscious.

anatomic equator: In ophthalmic usage, imaginary line around the circumference of the eyeball placed equidistant from the front and back surfaces (anterior and posterior poles) of the eyeball.

anesthetic: Drug that reduces or eliminates sensation, usually so that a surgical procedure may be performed without pain; **general a.** eliminates sensation by rendering the patient unconscious; usually administered systemically by intravenous injection or inhalation; **local a.** eliminates sensation in one area, usually administered by injection to either numb the tissue directly or to block the sensory nerves (called a *block*); **regional a.** another term for local a.; **topical a.** eliminates sensation in one area; usually administered by applying directly to the skin/tissue; tetracaine is a commonly used topical anesthetic in eyecare.

angiography: Evaluation of blood vessels following an injection of dye or radiopaque substance; in ophthalmology, generally referring to the examination of iris or retinal blood vessels; *see* fluorescein angiography.

angioid streaks: Red to brown streaks originating from the optic disk.

angioscotoma: Visual field defect caused by the shadow of a retinal blood vessel.

angle: 1. The point at which the upper and lower eyelids meet; *see also* canthus; 2. the area of the anterior chamber of the eye where the iris and cornea join (also called the *iridocorneal angle*); aqueous humor exits the eye through the angle, thus this structure is also called the *filtration angle;* specific tissues and structures that comprise the angle include the iris processes, corneoscleral junction, scleral sulcus, ciliary body, trabecular meshwork, and Schlemm's canal; 3. any one of several standard dimensions used to describe the optical system of the eye, specifically **alpha a.** angle formed at the eye's optical center by the optical and visual axes; **biorbital a.** angle formed by the axes of the two orbits; **gamma a.** angle formed at the eye's center of rotation by the optical and fixation axes; **kappa a.** angle formed at the eye's optical center by the pupillary and visual axes; **lambda a.** angle formed at the center of the eye's pupil by the optical and the visual axes; *see also* axis *and* optical center; **wetting a.** *see* wetting angle.

angle-closure glaucoma: *See* glaucoma.

angle of anomaly: Another term for *angle of deviation*.

angle of convergence: Angle formed by the eye's visual axis and a line drawn from the target object to a midpoint between the two eyes.

angle of deviation: Degree to which one eye is shifted from straight-ahead fixation when the fellow eye is fixed straight ahead; also called *angle of anomaly*.

angle of incidence: Angle formed by a ray of light that strikes (is "incident" to) an interface between two media, as measured from a line drawn perpendicular to the interface at the point where the light ray strikes.

angle of reflection: Angle formed by a ray of light reflected from the interface of two media, as measured from a line drawn perpendicular to the interface at the point from which the light ray is reflected.

angle of refraction: Angle formed by a ray of light that has crossed an interface between two substances and a line drawn perpendicular to the interface at the point where the light ray crosses.

angle-recession glaucoma: *See* glaucoma.

aniridia: The absence (sometimes congenital, though more frequently due to trauma in adults) of most or all of the iris.

aniseikonia: Condition in which the image size from an object is focused larger on one retina than on the other, resulting in distorted perception of spatial relations; *compare* iseikonia.

anisoaccommodation: General term for uneven accommodation in the two eyes.

anisochromatic: Color difference either between two or more objects or between different parts of the same object (as in an iris that is not of a uniform color); *see also* heterochromic; *compare* isochromatic.

anisocoria: Uneven size of pupils in the two eyes, usually reserved to describe more than a 1-mm difference in diameter; *compare* isocoria.

anisometropia: A difference between the refractive power of the two eyes, usually defined as more than a 1-diopter difference; *compare* isometropia.

anisophoria: Heterophoria in which there is an uneven latent deviation between the two eyes, depending on the direction of gaze.

anisopia: General term for unequal vision in the two eyes.

ankyloblepharon: Adhesion of the upper and lower eyelids.

annular: Ring-shaped.

annular cataract: *See* cataract.

annular keratitis: *See* keratitis.

annular scotoma: *See* scotoma.

annulus: General anatomic term for a ring-shaped structure.

annulus ciliaris: The outer portion of the ciliary body attached to the ora serrata.

annulus of Zinn: The ring of connective tissue attached to the orbit near the optic nerve, anchoring the rectus muscles of the eye (also called the *aponeurosis*).

anomalous or **abnormal retinal correspondence (ARC):** Condition in which parts of the images on each retina come to be linked in the brain's interpretation of the fused image even though they do not correspond to the same point in space, often occurring as a result of untreated strabismus; *compare* harmonious retinal correspondence.

anomalous trichromatism: *See* trichromatism.

anophthalmia, -os, -anopia: Congenital condition in which the eyeball is absent or only partially developed.

anopsia: Loss or suppression of vision, usually of only part of the visual field in just one eye.

anorthopia: General term for distortion of vision.

ANSI standards: Guidelines set forth in a document published by the American National Standards Institute (ANSI) that establish legal requirements for safety eyewear and other eyewear parameters.

antagonist: Muscle that opposes the contracting (agonist) muscle's action (eg, when the lateral rectus abducts the eye, the medial rectus is the antagonist); *compare* agonist.

anterior basal membrane: *See* Bowman's capsule/membrane.

anterior chamber (AC): Area within the eye formed by the structures in front of the iris and filled with aqueous humor; *compare* posterior chamber (which also contains aqueous humor).

anterior hyaloid membrane: *See* hyaloid membrane.

anterior pole (of the eye): Imaginary point on the front surface of the cornea centered over the pupil; *compare* posterior pole (of the eye).

anterior pole (of the lens): Point at the front and center of the crystalline lens; *compare* posterior pole (of the lens).

anterior segment (of the eye): General term usually describing the structures of the eye, including the lens and all structures anterior to the lens (thus including the anterior and posterior chambers); ophthalmic surgery is roughly divided into the categories of anterior segment (cornea, glaucoma, and cataract procedures) and posterior segment (retina and vitreous procedures); *compare* posterior segment (of the eye).

anterior synechia: Adhesion of the iris to the cornea; *see* synechiae; *compare* posterior synechiae.

anterior uveitis: Inflammation of the iris and ciliary body; *compare* iritis *and* posterior uveitis.

anterior vitrectomy: *See* vitrectomy.

antibacterial: Any substance/drug that destroys or inhibits bacteria.

antibiotic: Drug (derived from bacteria or fungi) used to destroy or inhibit microorganisms, and thus the disorders they cause.

anticholinesterase: Any substance or system that prevents cholinesterase from "cleaning" acetylcholine from receptor sites; they have a parasympathetic effect; an example is the drug eserine, which constricts the pupil and stimulates the ciliary muscle; *see also* cholinesterase *and* neurotransmitter.

antifungal: Any substance/drug that destroys or inhibits fungi.

antihistamine: Substance that blocks the release of histamine from mast cells, thus counteracting an allergic response.

antimetropia: Condition in which one eye is hyperopic while the fellow eye is myopic; also called *heterometropia*.

antimydriatic: Drug that prevents the pupil from dilating.

antiviral: Any substance/drug that destroys or inhibits viruses.

aphake: One in whom the lens of the eye is absent, either congenitally or following surgery.

aphakia: Absence of the lens of the eye; *see* cataract extraction.

aphakic: Adjective describing contact lenses or spectacles prescribed after removal of the crystalline lens of the eye; *see also* cataract extraction; *compare* phakic.

aphakic glaucoma: *See* glaucoma.

aphasia: The inability to verbalize.

aphotesthesia: Diminished response of the retina following excessive exposure to bright light.

apical clearance: 1. Distance between the back surface of a contact lens and the cornea; also called *vault*; 2. less commonly, distance between the cornea and the crystalline lens.

aplanatic, -ism: Property of an optical system such that it is free of the aberrations normally associated with spherical lenses.

aponeurosis: General term for the tendon that anchors a muscle; in the eye, the tendinous bundle that anchors the rectus muscles to the orbit (also called the *annulus of Zinn*).

apoptosis: General medical term for programmed cell death, a process by which cells continue to degenerate and cease functioning long after the initial injury or insult; in ophthalmic usage, usually referring to the progressive loss of retinal cells in glaucoma.

apostilb (abs): Unit of brightness; in ophthalmology, a measure of the brightness of a visual field test object.

apotripsis: Surgical excision of a corneal opacity.

applanation: Flattening of a normally rounded area, such as the cornea.

applanation tonometer: *See* tonometer.

applanometer: Another term for *applanation tonometer; see* tonometer.

aqueous flare: *See* flare.

aqueous fluid or **humor:** Clear, watery liquid (typically referred to simply as the aqueous) that fills the anterior or posterior chambers of the eye.

aqueous outflow: Process by which the aqueous humor is filtered out of the eye through the angle of the anterior chamber; *see also* angle, definition 2.

aqueous tap: Process of removing some aqueous from the anterior chamber through a needle.

arachnoid sheath: One of the membranes that surround the optic nerve.

arcuate keratotomy (AK): *See* keratotomy.

arcuate scotoma: *See* scotoma.

arcus juvenilis: Ring of fatty deposits around the edge of the cornea but not quite extending to the limbus, appearing in young or middle-aged patients with unusually high blood cholesterol levels or some systemic diseases.

arcus senilis: Ring of fatty deposits around the edge of the cornea but not quite extending to the limbus, appearing in elderly patients.

argon laser: *See* laser.

Argyll Robertson pupil (ARP): Condition in which a pupil constricts upon accommodation but does not react to varying direct or consensual light; usually associated with syphilis.

arterial circles of the iris: Two ring-shaped bands of vascular tissue in the iris: the inner or lesser circle is near the pupil and the major or greater circle is adjacent to the ciliary body.

arthro-ophthalmopathy: Degenerative disease that affects the joints and eyes; *see also* Sjögren's syndrome.

artificial tears: Man-made liquid formulated to simulate the composition of tear fluid, used in treating dry eye conditions.

aspheric, -al: Typically, in ophthalmic usage, a lens that focuses light along a meridian rather than to a point; aspheric lenses are used in spectacles, contact lenses, and intraocular lenses to correct astigmatism, to reduce peripheral distortion, or to provide a range of focusing power from near to far; *see also* cylinder *and* toric lens; *compare* spherical lens.

aspiration: In ophthalmic usage, suction applied by a surgical instrument, usually to remove fluid or particulate matter from the eye; *see* irrigation *and* aspiration.

aspiration flow rate: In phacoemulsification, the instrument setting that determines the maximum amount of fluid per unit of time (usually described in cubic centimeters per minute) that will flow through the eye into the instrument hand piece.

asteroid hyalosis: Small white bodies in the vitreous humor occurring most often in one eye, in the elderly, and in males more than females, usually with little effect on vision; they are composed of lipids and calcium.

asthenopia: Impairment of function such that the eye is weak and/or tires easily, possibly accompanied by ocular pain, diminished vision, and/or headache; **accommodative a.** asthenopia resulting from prolonged periods of accommodation (during reading or close work); **muscular a.** asthenopia attributable to tiring of the external ocular muscles; **nervous a.** asthenopia resulting from neurosis, characterized by eye fatigue and possibly constriction of the visual field; **tarsal a.** asthenopia attributable to pressure of the eyelids on the eye, which induces astigmatism.

astigmatic clock: Vision test target consisting of straight radial lines (like the spokes of a wheel); the patient reports which lines, if any, appear darker. (If using plus cylinder, the axis is parallel to the dark lines as the patient sees them; if using minus cylinder, the axis is perpendicular to the dark lines as the patient sees them.)

astigmatic or **arcuate keratotomy (AK):** Surgical correction of astigmatism by making partial-thickness, arcing incisions into specific areas of the cornea; *see also* keratotomy.

astigmatism (astig): Visual defect attributable to the presence of an elliptical (ie, egg- or football-shaped) rather than spherical shape in the refracting surfaces of the eye, resulting in the diffusion of light rays along a particular line (axis); **acquired a.** astigmatism resulting from some injury or insult to the eye; **against-the-rule a. (ATR)** astigmatism in which the steep axis is within 30 degrees of the horizontal; *compare* with-the-rule a.; **asymmetrical a.** astigmatism in which the steepest and flattest meridians are not 90 degrees from one another; **complex a.** combination of corneal and lenticular astigmatism in the same eye; **compound a.** astigmatism in which the flat and steep axes are either both hyperopic (compound hyperopic a.) or myopic (compound myopic a.); **corneal a.** astigmatism attributable to the shape of the refractive surface of the cornea; **direct a.** another term for *with-the-rule a.*; **hypermetropic** or **hyperopic a.** astigmatism; **inverse a.** another term for *against-the-rule a.*; **irregular a.** astigmatism in which the flat and steep axes are not at right angles or astigmatism resulting from variable curvature along a given meridian of the eye; **lenticular a.** astigmatism attributable to the shape of the refractive surfaces of the crystalline lens; **mixed a.** astigmatism in which one axis is hyperopic and the other is myopic; **myopic a.** astigmatism; **oblique a.** astigmatism occurring along the 45-degree or 135-degree meridians; *compare* against-the-rule a. *and* with-the-rule a.; **pathological a.** astigmatism that results from some disease; **physiologic a.** small degree of astigmatism occurring normally in virtually all eyes, usually unnoticed; **regular a.** astigmatism in which the curvatures of the flat and steep axes are uniform across the width of the eye and lie approximately at right angles to each other; **simple a.** astigmatism in which one focal line falls on the retina and the other falls behind the retina (simple hyperopia a.) or in front of the retina (simple myopia); **symmetrical a.** astigmatism in which the steepest and flattest meridians in opposite halves of the eye lie on a straight line through the center of the eye; **with-the-rule a. (WTR)** astigmatism in which the steep axis is within 30 degrees of the vertical (so named because it is the most common type of astigmatism found in the human eye); *compare* against-the-rule a.

astringent: Substance used to shrink tissues and stop any discharge.

atonic: General term for lack of muscle tone.

atonic ectropion: Condition in which weakness of the eyelid muscles results in the lid turning outward from the eye, exposing the conjunctiva.

atopic conjunctivitis: *See* conjunctivitis.

atopy: General term for condition marked by unusually high allergic sensitivity of many tissues throughout the body to a number of allergens.

attention reflex of the pupil: Change in the size of the pupil when fixation takes place.

audito-oculogyric reflex: Turning of the eye in the direction of startling noises.

autogenous keratoplasty or **autokeratoplasty:** Keratoplasty in which only the patient's own corneal tissues are used; *compare* homogenous keratoplasty.

automated lamellar keratoplasty (ALK or LK): Surgical procedure in which a microkeratome is used to make a corneal flap; this is followed by the flattening of the underlying cornea by microkeratome or laser (LASIK).

automated perimetry: *See* perimetry.

automated vitrectomy: *See* vitrectomy.

autonomic nervous system: Division of the nervous system that regulates the automatic processes of the body; its two branches are the sympathetic and parasympathetic nervous systems.

autorefractor or **automated refractor (AR):** Computerized instrument for objectively measuring the refractive power of the eye; *see* refractor.

A-V crossing: Situation in which the retinal arterioles press down on underlying veins that they cross over, reducing blood flow and causing A-V nicking.

A-V nicking: Situation in which the retinal arterioles and veins exhibit areas of compression, giving the appearance that a "nick" has been taken out of them; associated with hypertension.

axial hyperopia: *See* hyperopia.

axial length of the eye: Distance from the cornea's anterior to the surface of the retina along the principal axis of the eye.

axial myopia: *See* myopia.

axis: General term for the imaginary line passing through a solid body, representing a hypothetical axis around which the object could be rotated; any one of several standard reference lines used to describe the anatomy and optical system of the eye, specifically: **external a.** axis from anterior pole of the eye to the posterior pole; **internal a.** axis from the anterior pole of the eye to the point on the retina just opposite the posterior pole; **lens a.** axis from the anterior pole to the posterior pole of the crystalline lens; **optical a.** axis passing through the optical center of the eye and perpendicular to the plane of the crystalline lens; **principal a.** another term for *optical a.;* **pupillary a.** axis centered on and perpendicular to the plane of the pupil; **visual a.** axis along which light rays travel from an object to the macula (commonly referred to as the *line of sight*).

axometer: Instrument used for finding optical axes, especially as used in adjusting glasses.

axon: Filament extending from a nerve cell along which impulses are conducted away from the cell body toward the synapse; *see also* dendrite *and* synapse.

B

"B" measurement: The vertical eye size of a pair of spectacles, measured in millimeters from the top of the eyewire to the bottom; used in describing placement of the optical center or add position; *see also* boxing system.

B-scan: As used in ophthalmology, an ultrasound examination to create a cross-sectional view of the eye.

bacillary layer: Layer of column-like cells (rods and cones) in the retina.

back surface toric: *See* posterior toric.

back vertex power (BVP): Portion of the total refractive power imparted by the rear surface of a lens; *compare* front vertex power.

background diabetic retinopathy (BDR): *See* diabetic retinopathy.

bacterial conjunctivitis: *See* conjunctivitis.

bacterial endophthalmitis: *See* endophthalmitis.

bag: *See* capsule.

Bagolini lens: Lens with fine parallel lines across its width, used to evaluate retinal correspondence.

balanced salt solution: Mixture of water and salts (added to prevent electrolyte imbalance) used as an irrigating fluid in surgery.

ballast: *See* prism ballast.

band keratopathy/keratitis: *See* keratopathy.

bandage contact lens: *See* contact lens.

bar reader: Device placed between the reader and the page to block out different portions of a page for each eye; used in binocular vision diagnosis and divergence training.

Bard's sign: Phenomenon used to distinguish various types of nystagmus; patient with nystagmus is directed to follow finger motion across the field of view: in congenital nystagmus the rapid eye motions will decrease as the gaze shifts, while in organic nystagmus the motions increase.

barrel distortion: Bowed-out distortion of images that results from the steep curvature of spectacle lenses used to correct severe nearsightedness.

base curve (BC): General term for the curvature of the standard surface of a lens by which it is described; in spectacle and contact lenses, the base curve is measured on the less steep surface, most commonly the surface of the lens nearest the eye.

base-down (BD), base-in (BI), base-out (BO), and base-up (BU) prism: *See* prism.

basement membrane: General medical term for the layer of tissue underlying some epithelial cell layers.

basement membrane (of choroid): *See* Bruch's membrane.

basement membrane (of corneal epithelium): Thin membrane lying above Bowman's membrane to which the corneal epithelium adheres.

beam splitter: Optical device that uses a partially reflective mirror to divide light into two beams similar in appearance but of reduced intensity, typically to create two images for viewing or two laser beams for delivery.

bedewing (pronounced be-doó-ing): Appearance of dew-like deposits on the cornea (which is said to be "bedewed"); *see* guttata.

Behr's pupil: Dilation of the pupil resulting from a lesion far along the path of the optic nerve; because the two optic nerves cross, the dilated pupil will be on the opposite side of the body from the lesion.

Bell's palsy: Paralysis of the muscles of one side of the face due to inflammation of the facial nerve (CN VII), resulting in an inability to completely close the eyelids on that side; also called *facial palsy* or *seventh nerve palsy*.

Bell's phenomenon: Normal outward and upward rotation of the eyes that occurs when the lids are closed.

Benson's disease or **sign:** *See* asteroid hyalosis.

benzalkonium chloride: Preservative often used in contact lens care solutions and topical ophthalmic medications.

Berlin's edema: Severe swelling of the macula following a blow to the head, resulting in permanent loss of part of the visual field (also known as *commotio retinae*).

Berry's circle: Vision test target used to test stereopsis.

best corrected visual acuity (BCVA): Maximum visual acuity that can be achieved using corrective lenses to compensate for any refractive error; *see also* corrected visual acuity; *compare* best uncorrected visual acuity.

best uncorrected visual acuity (BUVA): Maximum visual acuity that is achieved without any corrective lenses; also called *uncorrected visual acuity*; *compare* best corrected visual acuity.

beta blockers: Class of drugs used to treat glaucoma by reducing aqueous production (eg, timolol, betaxolol, levobunolol); also called *adrenergic antagonists*.

biconcave lens: Lens that is concave (ie, hollow like a bowl) on both surfaces (also called a *minus lens*).

biconvex lens: Lens that is convex (ie, bulging outward) on both surfaces (also called a *plus lens*).

bifocal lens: Lens with two principal focal lengths (*see also* multifocal lens); a variety of such optical systems have been invented for vision correction (eg, bifocal spectacles or contact lenses used to correct presbyopia); there have also been bifocal intraocular lenses, but these represent only a small portion of the lenses in use.

bifoveal fixation: *See* fixation.

bilateral: Anatomic term describing something that appears or occurs on both sides or, in its specific ophthalmic use, both eyes of an individual; *compare* unilateral.

binocular: Said of visual properties or processes that involve both eyes working together; *compare* monocular; for binocular diplopia, binocular fixation, etc, see definitions under main words.

binocular microscope: Microscope that has two oculars (ie, eyepieces) for both the viewer's eyes, thus providing a three-dimensional view.

binocular ophthalmoscope: *See* ophthalmoscope.

binocular vision: A way of expressing the manner in which the two eyes work together; **grade 1 b.v.** vision in which there is simultaneous perception; **grade 2 b.v.** vision in which there is simultaneous perception as well as fusion; **grade 3 b.v.** highest quality of vision in which there is simultaneous perception, fusion, and stereopsis.

biomicroscope: *See* slit lamp.

bioptics: 1. Spectacles incorporating a telescopic lens system for use by low-vision patients. 2. in refractive surgery, the combination of two procedures to correct a large refractive error (eg, LASIK and phakic lens implantation).

bipolar cells: Retinal cells that bridge the light-perceiving bacillary layer and underlying nerve cells; *see also* retina.

bitoric lens: Contact lens that has a toric front surface to correct astigmatism and a toric back surface to prevent the lens from rotating, thus keeping it oriented in the proper axis.

Bjerrum's area: Area of retinal nerve fibers corresponding to the area between 12 and 20 degrees of the visual field; this is the most vulnerable area to damage by glaucoma.

Bjerrum's scotoma or **sign:** *See* scotoma.

black cataract: *See* cataract.

blanching of sclera: Whitening of the sclera.

blank: Unfinished spectacle or contact lens that has not yet been ground to its final refractive power.

blank size: Millimeter measurement of the lens blank required for a pair of spectacles; calculated by adding the effective diameter (ED) of the eyewire (with decentration, if any), plus 2 mm to allow for edging; *see also* effective diameter.

bleb: Soft-tissue space filled with fluid, most commonly in ophthalmic usage referring to a space created to receive drainage of aqueous fluid in glaucoma filtering surgery.

blend: Smoothing of the junctions between the zones of a contact lens to increase comfort and reduce prismatic aberration.

blephar-, -o-: Combining form meaning eyelid.

blepharitis: Inflammation of the eyelid, most often referring to the edge of the lid along which the eyelashes are located.

blepharoconjunctivitis: Inflammation of the conjunctiva and eyelid.

blepharophimosis: Condition in which the space between the eyelids is abnormally narrow.

blepharoplasty: General term for plastic surgical procedure of the eyelid(s) that can be reconstructive or cosmetic.

blepharoplegia: Paralysis of the eyelids.

blepharoptosis: *See* ptosis.

blepharorrhaphy: Suturing the eyelids together; also called *tarsorrhaphy*.

blepharospasm: Uncontrollable muscle spasm of the eyelid that may be strong enough to shut the eye; **essential b.** that which is not attributable to any defect of the structures of the eye or nerves.

blind spot: Area where the retina is joined to the optic nerve such that it forms a "funnel" of nerve cells that is not sensitive to light at its center; not usually noticed subjectively but readily detected even with the most simple visual field test; more properly called the *physiologic blind spot* to distinguish it from damaged areas of the retina.

blindness: Partial (as in the following terms) or total lack of the visual sense, more properly referred to as *amaurosis*; **color b.** colloquial term for impaired visual function at certain wavelengths of light (*see also* monochromatism); **hysterical b.** state of visual impairment that has an emotional rather than physical or physiological cause; **legal b.** state of visual impairment defined by public law or legal contract (eg, an insurance policy) precluding certain activities such as driving and qualifying individuals for certain tax or social service benefits; legal blindness is usually defined as best corrected Snellen's acuity of 20/200 or less in the better-seeing eye or visual field of 20 degrees or less; **night b.** *see* nyctalopia; **river b.** *see* onchocerciasis; *see also* count-finger vision, hand-motion vision, light perception vision, no light perception vision, *and* visual acuity.

blink reflex: Automatic response of eyelids to close when the cornea is touched.

blood-aqueous barrier, blood-eye barrier, or **blood-vitreous barrier:** Physiologic mechanisms that generally prevent passage of fluid or cells from the blood into the eye.

blowout fracture (of the orbit): Fracture in which the bones comprising the eye socket are disconnected and displaced outward from their normal position, if the fracture occurs in the orbital floor, extraocular muscles may herniate through the opening, limiting range of motion and causing diplopia.

blue-yellow perimetry: Colloquial term for visual field test in which the test targets are blue and yellow, which appears to enhance the ability of the test to locate field defects.

blur circle: *See* conoid of Sturm.

blur point: In testing visual acuity, the blur point is reached when the refractive power of a lens or prism can no longer be increased without causing vision to be blurred.

botulin or **botulinum (BTX):** Toxic substance produced by *Clostridium botulinum* bacteria, used in ophthalmology for treatment of blepharospasm and certain types of strabismus.

Bowman's capsule, layer, or **membrane:** Layer of the cornea lying above the corneal stroma and beneath the corneal epithelium; also called *anterior basal membrane.*

boxing system: Standardized way of measuring spectacle frames; *see also* "A" measurement, "B" measurement, *and* "C" measurement.

branch retinal artery (BRA): One of the small arteries that branch off the central retinal artery.

branch retinal artery occlusion (BRAO): Blockage of a branch retinal artery, usually in the temporal retina, impairing retinal blood flow but often resulting in no loss of vision or only minor visual field loss.

branch retinal vein (BRV): One of the small veins in the retina that drains into the central retinal vein.

branch retinal vein occlusion (BRVO): Blockage of blood flow in an area where a branch retinal vein is crossed by a branch retinal artery, resulting in retinal hemorrhage and a sudden blurring or loss of vision in part of the visual field.

break-up time (BUT): Length of time from the blink of an eye until the tear film evaporates, usually measured at the slit lamp using fluorescein dye.

bridge: Part of a spectacle frame front that crosses the nose and joins the two eyepieces.

bridle suture: Suture placed through the insertion of an extraocular muscle in order to give the surgeon control over the position of the eye.

Brightness Acuity Tester (BAT): *See* glare test.

Brown's syndrome: Condition, usually congenital but possibly as a result of trauma or arthritis, in which fibrous adhesions of the tendon sheath of the superior oblique muscle prevent the eye from looking upward in adduction.

Bruch's membrane: Innermost layer of the choroid to which the retinal pigment epithelium adheres.

brunescent: Brown; descriptive of very mature, dark cataracts.

buckling procedure: *See* scleral buckling procedure.

bulb: In ophthalmic usage, synonym for the eyeball.

bulbar conjunctiva: Portion of the conjunctiva that covers the eyeball, extending almost to the corneoscleral limbus; *compare* palpebral conjunctiva.

bullous keratopathy: Degeneration of the cornea; **pseudophakic b.k.** corneal degeneration attributable to implantation of an intraocular lens.

buphthalmia, -os: Condition in which the eye is abnormally large, most often used to describe pediatric eyes in which high intraocular pressure has distended the globe.

buttonhole: Complication of LASIK in which a thin, oblong hole forms in the center of the corneal flap.

C

C-loop lens: *See* intraocular lens.

"C" measurement: Horizontal measurement across the front of a pair of spectacles, including the "A" measurement of each eyewire plus the width of the bridge; also called the *datum line; see also* boxing system.

caloric nystagmus: *See* nystagmus.

canaliculitis: Inflammation of the tear duct, usually a result of infection or operative procedure.

canaliculus: Tear duct, more properly called *canaliculus nasolacrimalis;* plural: canaliculi.

canal of Schlemm: *See* Schlemm's canal.

candela (cd): Standard unit used in measurement of the intensity of light; the metric unit that replaced the "candle."

cannula: Tube used in surgery to perform irrigation or aspiration of fluids or to introduce smaller instruments into an incision.

can-opener capsulotomy: Surgical technique in which a series of small cuts are made in a circle around the periphery of the anterior lens capsule, which is then removed; *compare* capsulorrhexis.

canthotomy: Surgical procedure in which an incision is made into the area where the upper and lower eyelids meet.

canthus: Either of two angles formed by the meeting of the upper and lower eyelids; the one near the temple is called the *lateral canthus* and the one near the nose is called the *medial canthus;* plural: canthi.

capsular advancement: *See* advancement.

capsular opacification: Cloudiness of the lens capsule resulting from the spread of lens epithelial cells across the part of the capsule that remains after cataract extraction.

capsule: General medical term for the outer membrane surrounding an anatomic structure; most commonly in ophthalmic usage referring to the lens capsule, the transparent round sac containing the lens of the eye, attached at its periphery by the zonules to the ciliary body, often referred to as the capsular bag or simply "the bag;" **anterior c.** front portion of the capsule between the lens and the iris; **Bowman's c.** corneal layer between the stroma and epithelium; **posterior c.** rear portion of the capsule between the lens and the vitreous body; **Tenon's c.** thin, outermost membrane of the eye enclosing the entire globe except for the cornea.

capsulectomy: General term for surgical removal of a capsule.

capsulorrhexis: 1. Surgical procedure in which an anterior capsulotomy is made by puncturing, then grasping and tearing a hole in the capsule rather than by simply cutting it with a sharp instrument; *compare* can-opener capsulotomy; 2. the opening made in the capsule in this manner.

capsulotomy: 1. Surgical procedure to make an opening in a capsule, usually the lens capsule as the first step in extracapsular cataract extraction; 2. the opening made in the capsule in this manner; **anterior c.** surgical procedure to open the anterior capsule (or the opening itself), most commonly as one step in removal of a cataractous lens (*see also* can-opener c. *and* capsulorrhexis); **posterior c.** surgical procedure to open the posterior capsule (or the opening itself), often referring to the procedure performed with the Nd:YAG laser to open an opacified posterior capsule months or years after cataract extraction.

carbon dioxide laser: *See* laser.

carbonic anhydrase inhibitor (CAI): Class of glaucoma medications that act by reducing aqueous formation (eg, dorzolamide [topical], acetazolamide [oral]).

carcinoma (CA): Malignant growth arising from epithelial tissue.

cardinal points: Six points on the axis of an optical system that are used in describing its properties.

cardinal positions of gaze: *See* gaze.

caruncle: *See* lacrimal caruncle.

cataract: Area of opacification in ocular tissue that impedes the transmission of light rays to the retina; most commonly, the opacification of the lens that occurs as a natural consequence of aging, which is a leading cause of blindness in many parts of the world but surgically corrected on a wide scale (and with great success) in the developed world where ophthalmologic care is available; **after c.** opacification of the posterior lens capsule, following removal of a cataractous crystalline lens; the term is somewhat of a misnomer because the cataract does not actually recur; *see* capsular opacification; **annular c.** ring-shaped opacity of the lens in which the central lens remains clear; **axial c.** opacity located in the optical axis of the crystalline lens; **black c.** very mature (ie, advanced stage) cataract that is opaque black, very dense, and hard; **brunescent c.** very mature cataract that has a brownish appearance, often very dense and hard; **capsular c.** *see* capsular opacification; **complicated c.** another term for *secondary c.*; **congenital c.** cataract present at birth; **cortical c.** opacification of the lens cortex, usually in radial streaks or spokes, rather than the nucleus; **degenerative c.** opacification of ocular tissue that results from a degenerative change; *compare* developmental c.; **developmental c.** opacification of ocular tissue that results from a disturbance of normal development; **hypermature c.** progression of mature cataract to a state in which the lens begins to shrink and eventually soften, with harmful leakage of lens proteins; **intumescent c.** opacified lens that has swelled with absorbed fluid; **juvenile c.** cataract occurring in childhood; **lenticular c.** opacification of the crystalline lens; **mature c.** crystalline lens that has become opaque and exceedingly hard over a prolonged period of time; **morgagnian c.** progression of hypermature cataract in which the lens cortex is completely liquefied and the hard, opaque nucleus is no longer held stationary in the lens capsule; **nuclear c.** or **nuclear sclerotic (NS) c.** opacification of the center (nucleus) of the crystalline lens; **peripheral c.** opacification that is out of the optical axis and thus only minimally impairs vision; **polar c.** opacification located at the anterior or posterior pole of the crystalline lens; **posterior subcapsular c. (PSC)** opacification of the posterior part of the lens nucleus; **secondary c.** cataract associated with intraocular disorders, such as uveitis; the term is sometimes mistakenly applied to capsular opacification; **senile c.** cataract occurring in an elderly individual as a natural part of aging; **subcapsular c.** opacification of the inner surfaces of the lens capsule caused by overgrowth of epithelial cells; **traumatic c.** opacification of ocular tissue (especially the crystalline lens) resulting from a blow or penetrating injury to the eye, often quite rapid in onset and profound in extent.

cataract extraction (CE): General term for surgical procedures to remove the opacified crystalline lens of the eye; cataract extraction is essentially another term for crystalline lens removal; all such procedures have in common an incision into the anterior chamber of the eye, but there are many variations in the size of the incision, its location, and the instrumentation and technique used to remove the lens material; the eye immediately after cataract extraction is in a state known as *aphakia* (ie, without a lens), and an eye in which an intraocular lens has been implanted is said to be *pseudophakic* (ie, "false" lens); *see also* cryoextraction, extracapsular cataract extraction, intracapsular cataract extraction, *and* phacoemulsification.

cataractogenic: Causing or facilitating the formation of a cataract.

cataractous: Ocular tissue that is like or affected by cataract.

cat's eye pupil: Condition in which the pupil is a narrow vertical slit.

cautery: Use of heat to burn or scar tissue; can also refer to similar use of electric current, cold (*see* cryo-), or chemicals.

cavitation: In ophthalmic usage, a phenomenon in which the ultrasonically vibrating phacoemulsification tip creates microscopic areas of intense turbulence that pulverizes lens material.

cell: In ophthalmic usage, the appearance of white blood cells in the anterior chamber as a result of inflammation, most often following surgery or trauma; *see also* flare.

cell and flare (C/F): In ophthalmic usage, usually the appearance of white blood cells in the anterior chamber accompanied by the presence of protein particles in the aqueous humor, indicating intraocular inflammation, usually after surgery or trauma.

cellophane maculopathy: *See* epiretinal membrane.

central fixation: *See* fixation.

central fusion: *See* fusion.

central nervous system (CNS): The half of the nervous system controlled by the brain and spinal cord.

central retinal artery: One of the main blood vessels bringing blood into the retina from the ophthalmic artery.

central retinal artery occlusion: Blockage of the central retinal artery resulting in sudden, permanent loss of vision across a wide area of the visual field.

central retinal vein: Major vein that drains blood from the retina, exiting the eye in the area of the optic nerve.

central retinal vein occlusion: Blockage of the central retinal vein resulting in retinal hemorrhage and sudden loss of vision, usually involving the central visual field.

central scotoma: *See* scotoma.

central serous chorioretinopathy (CSC): Condition similar to central serous retinopathy, except with greater involvement of the choroid; *see* central serous retinopathy.

central serous retinopathy (CSR): Condition in which there is swelling and elevation of retinal tissues in the area of the macula, sometimes progressing to the point of detachment, that causes a perceptible but usually not permanent visual field loss.

central suppression: Action of the brain to ignore the portion of the image in the center of the visual field.

centrocecal scotoma: *See* scotoma.

chalazion: Chronic granuloma of the eyelid resulting from blockage and inflammation of a meibomian gland; *see also* meibomian cyst; *compare* hordeolum.

chatter: In ophthalmic usage, undesirable phenomenon in phacoemulsification in which the crystalline lens rapidly vibrates on the instrument tip as it is simultaneously attracted by aspiration and repelled by the vibration of the tip.

chemosis: Swelling of the conjunctiva; adjective: chemotic.

chiasm: General anatomic term for an intersection (from the Greek letter chi, which is written as X); *see* optic chiasm.

chlorolabe: Visual pigment present in the "green" retinal cones that absorbs light in the green frequencies (around 540 nm); one of three visual pigments; *see also* cyanolabe, erythrolabe, *and* trichromatism.

choked disk: *See* papilledema.

cholinergic: Refers to substances that activate the parasympathetic nervous system; also called *parasympathomimetic*; pilocarpine is a cholinergic drug; *compare* adrenergic.

cholinesterase: Enzyme that "cleans up" the neurotransmitter acetylcholine; blocking its action allows the neurotransmitter to have a prolonged effect; *see* anticholinesterase.

chondroitin sulfate: Component of some viscoelastic materials.

choriopathy: Noninflammatory disease of the choroid.

chorioretinal: Of or involving the choroid and retina.

choroid: Highly vascular tissue layer lying under the retina, merging at the angle of the anterior chamber with the ciliary body and the iris (all three areas comprise the uvea).

choroidal detachment: Separation of the choroid from the sclera, usually as a result of injury.

choroidal neovascular membrane: Network of vascular tissue resulting from choroidal neovascularization.

choroidal neovascularization (CNV): Condition in which new, abnormal blood vessels grow into the choroid beneath the retinal pigment epithelium.

choroidal nevus: Small, well-defined area of benign pigmentation or vascularization in the choroid.

choroideremia: Sex-linked hereditary condition in which the retinal pigment epithelium and choroid begin to degenerate in the first few months or years after birth; in males it eventually leads to blindness but in females it rarely causes significant vision loss.

choroiditis: Inflammatory disease of the choroid.

chromatic aberration: Uneven focusing of an optical system such that white light is partially or completely broken down into its component colors.

chronic: In medical usage, denoting the long-term or nonemergency; *compare* acute.

cicatrix: Scar tissue (adjective: cicatricial); some cases of ectropion and entropion are described as cicatricial, and some glaucoma operations construct what is known as a *cicatricial filter*.

cilia: Plural of cilium.

ciliaris: *See* ciliary muscle.

ciliary: 1. Of or related to the eyelashes; 2. of or related to the ring-shaped structure joining the iris and choroid; *see* ciliary body.

ciliary arteries: Several branches of the ophthalmic artery that carry blood to every anatomic structure of the eye except the inner part of the retina.

ciliary body: Ring-shaped structure joining the iris to the choroid and containing the ciliary muscle and ciliary processes.

ciliary muscle: Ring-shaped muscle in the ciliary body; it contracts when stimulated by a near target; *see also* accommodation.

ciliary nerves: Any of several nerve fiber bundles that carry nerve impulses to the pupillary sphincter and ciliary muscle, as well as from the cornea (short ciliary nerves), or that carry impulses either to the pupillary dilator muscle or sensory impulses from the cornea, iris, and ciliary body (long ciliary nerves).

ciliary processes: Finger-shaped extensions of the ciliary body that produce aqueous humor and provide an attachment for the zonules that support the lens capsule.

ciliary spasm: Painful contractions of the ciliary body due to some pathologic condition (eg, iritis) or drug (eg, pilocarpine).

ciliary sulcus: Groove formed by the junction of the ciliary body and iris; posterior chamber intraocular lenses are sometimes placed into the sulcus when implantation into the lens capsule is not possible.

ciliary veins: Any of several veins that drain blood from the major structures of the eye.

cilium: Term for the eyelashes; single: cilia.

circle of Zinn: *See* annulus of Zinn.

circumduction of the eye: Circular "rolling" of the eye, applicable to voluntary and involuntary movement.

clear lensectomy: Refractive surgical procedure to correct large degrees of nearsightedness by removing the crystalline lens.

clock dial: *See* astigmatic clock.

closed-angle glaucoma: *See* glaucoma.

CMV (cytomegalovirus) retinitis: *See* retinitis.

cobalt blue filter: Light filter placed on the slit lamp light source to induce fluorescence of topical fluorescein dye for corneal examination; *see also* exciter filter.

coherent light: Light in which all of the component waves are in phase as in a laser beam; *see also* laser *and* phase.

collarette: 1. Crusting at the base of an eyelash in blepharitis; 2. border between pupillary and ciliary zones of the iris, visible on the anterior surface of the iris as a line of transitional color about 1.5 mm from the edge of the pupil.

collyrium: General term for an eyewash.

coloboma: Partial absence of or gap in ocular structures, as in retinal coloboma, iris coloboma, etc, usually in the lower half of the eye and usually as a result of incomplete fusion of fetal tissue; **atypical c.** coloboma in the upper half of the eye.

color: Subjective perception of the varying wavelengths of light.

color adaptation: *See* adaptation.

color blindness: *See* blindness *and* deuteranopia.

columnar layer: Cell layer of the retina consisting of column-like cells (rods and cones); also called the *bacillary layer*.

comitant: Another term for concomitant.

comitant strabismus: *See* strabismus.

commotio retinae: *See* Berlin's edema.

compliance: Meeting guidelines; may refer to the patient (as in compliance with treatment programs) or to the physician/practitioner (as in compliance with laws and other specifications).

compound astigmatism, compound hyperopic astigmatism, or **compound myopic astigmatism:** *See* astigmatism.

computerized tomography (CT or **CAT) scan:** Imaging technique using ionizing radiation to visualize inner structures of the body; in ophthalmology used to evaluate fractures, inflammation, or tumors; *compare* magnetic resonance imaging.

concave: Having a curved, indented surface, like the inside of a bowl; *compare* convex.

concave lens: Lens with a concave surface that causes parallel rays of light to diverge and thus can be used to correct myopia; *see also* minus lens; **double c.l.** lens that has two concave surfaces.

concavoconvex lens: Lens that has one concave and one convex surface.

concomitant: Adjective describing a constant, uniform relationship between the lines of sight of the two eyes regardless of the direction of gaze, usually referring to strabismus; *compare* incomitant; *see* strabismus.

concomitant strabismus: Another term for comitant strabismus; *see* strabismus.

cone: Term used in ophthalmic applications to geometrically describe anatomic structures and optical properties; **distraction c.** white crescent-shaped area sometimes seen on funduscopy in myopic eyes; **myopic c.** staphyloma at the posterior pole of the eye; **ocular c.** the eyeball and its sheath of muscle, blood vessels, and nerves, approximately conical in shape.

cone cells or **retinal cones:** One of two types of light-sensitive cells in the retina (rods are the other type); often simply referred to as *cones*, they are concentrated in the macula and function in the discrimination of color and fine detail mainly in the central field of view under lighted conditions; *compare* rod cells.

confrontation field test: Gross method for measuring the approximate extent of the visual field; the examiner sits facing the test subject and holds a target far to the subject's side, then brings it slowly into the field of view; the subject reports when the object becomes visible.

congenital: Present at birth; *compare* infantile, juvenile, *and* senile.

congruous: Similar in form.

congruous field defect: Visual field defects of similar shape in both eyes.

congruous hemianopia: Loss of half the visual field in each eye in which the field defects are the same size, shape, and location.

conjunctiva (conj): Ocular tissue lining the inner surface of the eyelids (ie, **palpebral c.**), which folds in to join with the tissue covering the sclera (ie, **bulbar c.**); the "pocket" of the fold is called the *cul de sac*; **limbal c.** edge of the conjunctiva overlying the sclera near its transition zone into the cornea.

conjunctival injection: Condition in which the conjunctiva is red, swollen, and engorged with dilated blood vessels.

conjunctivitis: General term for inflammation of the conjunctiva; colloquially known as *pink eye*; **allergic c.** conjunctivitis resulting from an allergic reaction, either to airborne allergens or substances (such as topical medications) placed into the eye; **atopic c.** conjunctivitis occurring as one manifestation of systemic allergy (atopia); **bacterial c.** conjunctivitis resulting from an infection of the surface tissues of the eye; **c. of newborn** purulent conjunctivitis of an infant less than 2 weeks old; **follicular c.** appearance of tiny clear or yellow sacs of lymphocytes and inflammatory cells on the conjunctiva after prolonged irritation, often as a result of viral infection; **giant papillary c. (GPC)** condition in which wart-like protrusions (ie, papillae) appear on the inside of the eyelid accompanied by mucus discharge; **herpetic c.** conjunctivitis resulting from an infection with herpes virus; **inclusion c.** inflammation of the conjunctiva due to presence of Chlamydia organisms; also called *ophthalmia neonatorum*; **vernal c.** chronic allergic conjunctivitis that occurs in both eyes during warm weather; **viral c.** conjunctivitis resulting from an infection with a virus.

conoid of Sturm: Geometric representation of light refracted through a lens that is spherical along one axis and cylindrical along another.

consecutive: In ophthalmic usage, describing a condition (usually unwanted) that results after surgery (eg, consecutive hyperopia is an adverse result of radial keratotomy to correct myopia).

consensual pupillary reflex: *See* pupillary reflex.

consent: *See* informed consent.

constant exotropia: *See* exotropia.

contact angle: Another term for wetting angle.

contact lens (CL or **CR):** 1. Vision-correcting lens placed directly on the cornea of the eye; *see also* aspheric lens, bifocal lens, multifocal lens, *and* toric lens; **bandage c.l.** lens used for therapeutic purposes (usually to protect the cornea or deliver medication following surgery or trauma) rather than to correct vision; **corneal c.l.** contact lens designed to rest upon the cornea rather than extending onto the sclera; **daily wear (DW) c.l.** contact lens that is approved for wear during waking hours only and is to be removed every day; **disposable c.l.** soft contact lens that is worn for a specified time then discarded and replaced with a fresh lens; **extended wear (EW) c.l.** contact lens that is approved for wear during sleep; **fitting c.l.** lens used to check for correct fit on patient before a contact lens prescription is given or lenses dispensed; **gas-permeable (GP) c.l.** modern contact lens composed of polymers formulated to transmit oxygen; **hard c.l.** contact lens composed of polymethylmethacrylate (rarely used now); **keratoconus c.l.** rigid contact lens designed to correct and retard keratoconus; **rigid c.l.** contact lens made of relatively inflexible material (vs. "soft"); term usually refers to gas-permeable contacts; **scleral c.l.** contact lens designed so that its periphery rests on the sclera rather than the cornea; **soft (S) c.l.** modern contact lens made from silicone or water-containing hydroxyethylmethacrylate (HEMA); **trial c.l.** another term for fitting c.l.; 2. hand-held lens system, usually incorporating prisms and/or mirrors, placed on the cornea to provide a view inside the eye or to focus laser energy for delivery into the eye.

contraindication: Reason(s) why a treatment or procedure should *not* be done.

contrast: Property of an image such that it has bright and dark areas; the relative brightness of the various components can be measured in comparison to each other or against a reference gray scale.

contrast sensitivity: The ability to distinguish fine gradations of brightness, often diminished under conditions of glare especially in the presence of a cataract and other ocular pathology.

contrast sensitivity test (CST): Vision test target consisting of patterns of lines (sinusoidal gratings) of various densities: the test subject is asked to describe the orientation of the lines (vertical, horizontal, oblique); acuity is the most closely spaced lines that the subject can correctly discern; the basis for the test is that the traditional eye chart is high contrast, giving a measurement of better acuity than actually exists, especially in the presence of cataracts and other pathology.

convergence: 1. In optics, the gathering together of parallel light rays to a point of focus after passing through a plus lens; 2. in ophthalmic usage, coordinated action of ocular muscles that draws both eyes inward to fixate upon the same point in space (also called *positive convergence*); the processes of convergence and accommodation normally are linked; **accommodative c.** convergence stimulated by and working in conjunction with accommodation; **fusional c.** convergence operating to keep an image focused upon the foveae of both eyes; **near point of c.** point at which the eyes can no longer maintain fixation together on an approaching near object and one eye drifts out (also called *maximum convergence*); **negative c.** *see* divergence; **positive c.** synonym for convergence; **tonic c.** degree of convergence maintained by the tone of the ocular muscles.

convergence excess: Condition in which the eyes "overshoot" (ie, move inward too much) during near vision.

convergence insufficiency: Condition in which the eyes fail to turn inward enough to achieve fusion during near vision.

convergent lens: *See* plus lens.

convergent strabismus: *See* esotropia; *see also* strabismus.

convex: Having a rounded, protruding surface, like a globe; *compare* concave.

convex lens: Lens with a convex surface that causes parallel rays of light to converge and thus can be used to correct hyperopia; *see also* plus lens; **double c.l.** lens that has two convex surfaces.

convexoconcave lens: Lens that has one convex and one concave surface.

core-, -o-: Combining form meaning pupil.

corectopia: Condition in which the pupil is not in the center of the iris.

cornea (K): Clear structure at the front of the eye overlying the iris; it imparts the greatest focusing power of all the ocular media; composed (from outer- to innermost) of the epithelium, Bowman's membrane, the stroma, Descemet's membrane, and the endothelium; the cornea joins the sclera at the limbus and consists of similar tough, fibrous tissue; *see also* words beginning with the root kerat-, meaning cornea.

corneal abrasion: Injury in which tissues are scraped from an area on the surface of the cornea, usually involving the corneal epithelium but possibly extending more deeply.

corneal astigmatism: *See* astigmatism.

corneal bedewing: Dew-like beads on the surface of the cornea, usually visible only under magnification; *see* guttata.

corneal button: Piece of corneal tissue, either full thickness (for penetrating keratoplasty) or partial thickness (a lamellar keratoplasty), intended for use as a graft.

corneal cap: Complication of LASIK surgery in which the corneal flap detaches; *see also* flap.

corneal decompensation: Condition in which chronic failure of the corneal endothelium to maintain the proper water content of the corneal stroma results in swelling, clouding, and degeneration of the cornea.

corneal dellen: Small concavities at the outer edges of the cornea that sometimes appear after ocular surgery.

corneal dystrophy: General term for hereditary condition in which there is defective development or degeneration of corneal tissue; **endothelial c.d.** condition, possibly worse in one eye than the other but always present bilaterally, in which guttata appear in the corneal endothelium, eventually resulting in loss of vision due to corneal edema as normal endothelial function is impaired; *see also* guttata; **Fuchs' c.d.** progressive degeneration of the cornea related to dysfunction of the corneal epithelium; **map-dot-fingerprint (MDF) c.d.** condition in which small concentric dots and lines with the appearance of a map or fingerprint appear in the corneal epithelium.

corneal ectasia: Outward bulging of the cornea that occurs when corneal tissue is thinned or weakened.

corneal edema: Condition in which the cornea swells with water and becomes cloudy; almost always a result of damage to the corneal endothelium.

corneal endothelium: Innermost layer of the cornea, only one cell thick, that acts to pump excess water out of the cornea; these cells are quite delicate and do not regenerate if damaged.

corneal epithelium: Outermost layer of the cornea, only one cell thick, that regenerates rapidly if damaged or even if the whole layer is removed (as in certain ophthalmic procedures).

corneal erosion: Loss of the corneal epithelium over some or all of the area of the cornea; **recurrent c.e.** chronic condition in which erosion periodically occurs due to inadequate adhesion of regenerated epithelium to its basement membrane.

corneal guttata: *See* guttata *and* endothelial corneal dystrophy *under* corneal dystrophy.

corneal hydrops: Accumulation of aqueous fluid within the cornea as a result of the loss of tissue integrity of the corneal endothelium and Descemet's membrane.

corneal lathing: Another term for keratomileusis.

corneal map: Another term for corneal topography.

corneal melting: Condition in which layers of the cornea degenerate and slough off due to an inflammatory process.

corneal reflection pupillometer (CRP): Device used to measure pupillary distance by using the reflection of the instrument's light on the cornea; gives binocular and monocular measurements; *see also* pupillary distance.

corneal reflex: *See* blink reflex.

corneal staining: Method of evaluating the cornea (usually with the slit lamp) using dye; fluorescein dye will pool into any corneal defects or under contact lenses and glow bright green when observed with a cobalt blue light; the pattern of fluorescein staining often assists in diagnosis; rose bengal stains any degenerated or dead corneal epithelium.

corneal stroma: Transparent connective tissue making up the central layer of the cornea.

corneal topography: Technique in which an image projected onto the cornea is analyzed by a computer to obtain a representation of the shape of the corneal surface and thus an indication of its refractive power; also known as *videokeratography*.

corneal transplant: *See* keratoplasty.

corneal ulcer: Loss of tissue from the surface of the cornea due to a disease process, often an infection.

corneoscleral: Of or involving the cornea and sclera.

corneoscleral junction or **spur:** *See* scleral spur.

corrected visual acuity (Va$_{cc}$): Visual acuity measured with the patient's current corrective lenses in place (ie, no attempt is made to improve further vision optically); *compare* best corrected visual acuity *and* uncorrected visual acuity.

correction: In ophthalmic usage, spectacles or contact lenses prescribed to counteract myopia, hyperopia, astigmatism, or any other ametropia.

correspondence: *See* retinal correspondence.

cortex: In ophthalmic usage, the soft outer portion of the crystalline lens of the eye; **visual c.** area of the occipital lobe of the brain that receives visual input.

cortical attachments: Areas in which the nucleus and cortex of the crystalline lens adhere together.

corticosteroids: Substances used to reduce inflammation; topical steroid drugs used in ophthalmology include prednisone, dexamethasone, and fluorometholone; topical steroids are sometimes combined with antibiotics to fight infection as well; side effects in the eye can include increased intraocular pressure; *compare* nonsteroidal anti-inflammatory drugs.

cotton-wool spots (CWS): Small areas of the retinal nerve fiber layer that have lost their blood supply and become wispy white spots with no clear borders; also called *soft exudates* although technically they are not exudates; *see also* retinal exudates.

couching: Obsolete treatment for cataract in which the whole lens of the eye was detached and pushed out of the visual axis, usually accomplished with a needle inserted into the anterior chamber of the eye.

count-finger vision: Very low level of visual acuity in which no greater detail can be perceived than the number of fingers held before the eyes; *see also* hand-motion vision, light perception vision, no light perception vision, *and* visual acuity.

coupling agent: In ophthalmology, a clear, thick substance used to cushion a lens (eg, goniolens) or probe (eg, B scan) where it contacts ocular tissues.

cover test: Test to determine the presence of phoria or tropia; there are several types but all involve having the subject fixate on a target while the examiner covers an eye and observes for any movement; if there is no movement, the patient is orthophoric; **alternate c.t.** cover test performed by quickly moving the occluder from one eye to the other so that there is no time for binocular fixation to occur; used to detect the presence and direction of deviation but cannot distinguish between aphoria and tropia; also called *cross cover test;* **cover-uncover test** cover test performed by covering then uncovering one eye; used to distinguish between tropia and phoria and direction of deviation; **prism and alternate c.t. (PACT)** or **prism and c.t.** use of prisms in conjunction with alternate cover test in order to measure the amount of deviation.

cranial nerve(s) (CN): Twelve pairs of nerves (motor, sensory, and mixed) that originate in the brain, designated both by Roman numerals (I to XII) and names; six of them affect vision either directly or indirectly; the optic nerve is CN II; *see* Appendix 4.

crazing: In ophthalmic usage, the appearance of a network of fine lines or cracks on a lens, most often a contact lens.

cribrosa: Another term for lamina cribrosa.

cross cylinder: Lens comprised of two cylindrical components of the same power, one plus and one minus, superimposed at right angles to each other, used to measure astigmatism; also called *Jackson cross cylinder lens.*

cross fixation: Condition in which the left eye becomes dominant in gaze toward the extreme right and the right eye becomes dominant in gaze toward the extreme left.

crossed diplopia: Another term for heteronymous diplopia.

crossing changes: Another term for AV crossing.

cryo-: Combining form meaning cold, used in medical terminology to describe treatments or surgical procedures involving very low temperatures (usually several hundred degrees below zero).

cryoextraction: Technique of intracapsular cataract extraction in which the lens capsule and its contents are frozen to the tip of a surgical instrument (ie, cryoprobe) and removed as a unit; now largely abandoned in the United States but still performed by many surgeons around the world; *see also* cataract extraction, extracapsular cataract extraction, intracapsular cataract extraction, *and* phacoemulsification.

cryopexy: Surgical procedure that attempts to fix a tissue into place by application of extreme cold (most commonly in ophthalmic usage, a detached retina against the choroid).

cryophake: Instrument used in cataract cryoextraction.

cryoprobe: General term for instrument used in cryosurgery.

cryoretinopexy: *See* retinopexy.

cryosurgery or **cryotherapy:** General term for application of extreme cold to tissue.

crystalline lens: Proper term for the natural lens of the eye (usually called simply *the lens*), consisting of a soft outer cortex and hard nucleus in the center; use of the full term crystalline lens is helpful as a distinction from manufactured lenses for vision correction.

cul de sac: General anatomic term for a sac with only one opening (from French for "bottom of the bag"); in ophthalmic usage, the sac formed by the bulbar and palpebral conjunctivae; *see also* conjunctiva.

cup: General term referring to a depression; **glaucomatous c.** *see* cupping; **physiologic c.** in ophthalmic usage, the normal slight depression at the center of the optic nerve.

cup-to-disk ratio (c/d): Measure of the proportion of damaged area (ie, cup) to visually functional area (ie, disk) of the retina, representing the relative progression of glaucomatous damage; *see also* glaucoma.

cupping: Sign of glaucomatous damage in which the optic disk is affected by an area of increasing concavity, representing nonfunctioning retinal cells.

cyanolabe: Visual pigment present in the "blue" retinal cones that absorb light in the blue frequencies (around 440 nm); one of three visual pigments: *see also* chlorolabe, erythrolabe, *and* trichromatism.

cycl-, -o-: Combining form meaning circle or ring; in ophthalmic usage, the iris and/or ciliary body.

cyclitic membrane: Formation of fibrous tissue in the anterior part of the vitreous body as a result of severe inflammation of the ciliary body.

cyclitis: Inflammation of the ciliary body.

cyclocryotherapy: Application of very low temperatures to the ciliary body performed in an attempt to decrease the production of aqueous fluid by the ciliary processes as a treatment for glaucoma.

cyclodestruction: General term for glaucoma surgical procedures that destroy portions of the ciliary body (as with extreme cold, laser energy, or other means) in order to decrease the production of aqueous fluid.

cyclodialysis: Largely abandoned glaucoma surgical procedure in which the root of the iris is detached from the ciliary body so that aqueous fluid may pass more easily out of the anterior chamber and thus reduce intraocular pressure.

cycloduction: Rotation of one eye around its visual axis (anterior-posterior pole); also called *cyclotorsion; compare* cyclovergence.

cycloplegia: Paralysis of the ciliary muscle in which the eye does not accommodate in response to the usual stimuli.

cyclovergence: Rotation of both eyes around their visual axes (anterior-posterior poles); if the right eye rotates clockwise, the left eye rotates counterclockwise and vice versa; *compare* cycloduction.

cylinder (cyl): 1. In optics, a lens that is flat along one axis and circularly curved along the perpendicular axis or the property of a lens that is relatively flat along one axis and more curved along the perpendicular axis; 2. in refraction, the component of refractive error that can be corrected with a cylindrical lens (roughly synonymous with astigmatism); *compare* sphere; **minus c.** refracting surface of a lens in which the lens material is fashioned into the concave reverse of a cylindrical shape (ie, as if a cylinder had been carved out of the lens and discarded); **plus c.** refracting surface of a lens in which the lens material is fashioned into the convex shape of a cylinder.

cystoid macular edema (CME): Swelling of the central focusing area of the retina, typically as a result of trauma or as a complication of ophthalmic surgery.

cystotome: Surgical instrument for cutting a sac; most often in ophthalmic usage, instrument for cutting into the lens capsule.

cytomegalovirus (CMV) retinitis: *See* retinitis.

dacry-, -o-: Combining form meaning tear fluid; *see also* combining forms beginning with lacri-.

dacryocyst: *See* nasolacrimal sac.

dacryocystitis: Inflammation of the nasolacrimal sac, usually because of an infection and blocked nasolacrimal duct.

dacryocystorhinostomy (DCR): Procedure in which an opening between the dacryocyst and the nasal passage is created or reopened.

dark adaptation: *See* adaptation.

datum line: Another term for "C" measurement.

decentration: General term for misalignment; in ophthalmic usage, usually referring to displacement of a lens (spectacle, contact, or intraocular) out of the visual axis.

decongestant: Substance used to reduce swelling and blood accumulation in an area; in ophthalmic usage, a drug that reduces ocular redness.

degenerative cataract: *See* cataract.

degenerative myopia: *See* myopia.

dehiscence: General medical term for a splitting open of tissue, often as a result of fibrosis in the course of healing of a traumatic or surgical wound; in ophthalmic usage, typically referring to splitting of retinal tissue or breakage of the lens zonular fibers.

dellen: *See* corneal dellen.

dendrite: Short filaments of a nerve cell body that receive impulses from other nerve cells (via the axons of those cells); *see also* axon *and* synapse.

dendritic: Describing a tree-like shape; used often in ophthalmic terminology to describe lesions on the cornea that have a branched appearance (eg, as in dendritic keratitis).

depth of field: Space in front of and behind an object of regard in which other objects can also be clearly seen; the depth of field is typically very shallow for nearby objects and deeper for very distant objects; typically of consideration in photography.

depth perception: The ability to discern the relative distance of objects within the field of view, made possible by the varying degrees of convergence necessary to focus upon objects at varying distances from the observer; present even when binocular vision and fusion are not achieved; *compare* stereopsis.

dermatochalasis: Condition in which the skin of the eyelid sags, sometimes enough to overlap the lid margin and block vision.

Descemet's membrane: Inner tissue layer of the cornea to which the corneal endothelium adheres.

detachment: Separation of tissue layers that are normally attached; in ophthalmic usage, most commonly referring to the retina or choroid; *see also* retinal detachment *and* vitreous detachment.

deutan: Color vision defect involving the green color mechanism and linked to the X chromosome; this is the most common form of color blindness.

deuteranomaly: Partial impairment of the green color mechanism resulting in poor red/green discrimination, although red is normally vivid.

deuteranopia, -opsia: Severe lack of the green color mechanism; red and yellow-green both look orange; red-orange, orange, and yellow are all the same strong red-orange color; magenta and green are gray tones; blue-green to purple are various confusing shades of blue.

deviation: In ophthalmic usage, a turning of the eye from the point of fixation; **convergent d.** *see* esotropia; **dissociated vertical d.** deviation in which either eye drifts upward when it is occluded; **divergent d.** *see* exotropia; **primary d.** where an ocular muscle is paralyzed, the deviation that exists when the nonparalyzed eye is fixating; **secondary d.** where an ocular muscle is paralyzed, the deviation that exists when the affected eye is forced to fixate (typically the primary d. is less than the secondary d.); **skew d.** a vertical strabismus caused by an anomaly in the brainstem or cerebellum.

dextro-: Prefix describing structures or processes appearing or occurring toward the right; referring to the right eye in ophthalmic usage, as in the phrase oculus dexter (OD); *compare* sinistro-.

diabetic retinopathy (DR): Ocular effect(s) of diabetes mellitus, characterized by edema, bleeding, and neovascularization of the retina, with progressive loss of vision if left untreated; laser therapy is currently used in treatment; **background d.r. (BDR)** earlier stage of DR characterized by small hemorrhages and macular edema; **proliferative d.r. (PDR)** severe stage of DR in which neovascularization, large hemorrhages, and ischemia occur.

dialysis: In ophthalmic usage, the separation of connected tissues or structures.

dichromatism: Condition in which only two of the three retinal cone pigments are present; *compare* achromatism, monochromatism, *and* trichromatism.

diffraction: Property of light attributable to its wave-like nature: light passing through a very narrow opening (about the same width as the wavelength of the light) is bent from its original path; theoretically, diffraction provides an alternative optical system to refraction for artificial lens design.

diffractive multifocal lens: Optical system that attempts to use diffraction in order to impart two or more focal points to incoming light, one "fundamental" focus provided by conventional refractive optics and the other(s) provided by diffraction.

diffuse illumination: In slit lamp biomicroscopy, the use of nonfocused, scattered light to provide a view of the whole eye and its adnexa, often for photography.

diffuser: Filter for the light source of an optical instrument that scatters light without changing its color, thereby reducing reflections that can occur with point sources of illumination.

digital tonometry: Method for estimating intraocular pressure by judging the eyeball's resistance to a finger pressed against it.

dilation or **dilatation:** General term for widening of an opening; in ophthalmic usage, the widening of the pupil in dim light or as a result of pharmaceuticals (more properly called *mydriasis*); dilation must be induced in order to perform certain intraocular examinations and surgical procedures.

dimer: A compound that is formed by the joining of two like molecules; *see also* excimer laser *under* laser.

diode laser: *See* laser.

diopter (D): 1. Measure of the focusing power of a lens, defined as the reciprocal of the focal length measured in meters; for example, a lens that focuses light from a very distant object ("infinity") to a point 1 m behind the lens has a power of 1 D, whereas a lens that focuses light at 2 m has a power of 0.5 D; 2. by analogy, degrees of myopia (designated as minus diopters) or hyperopia (designated as plus diopters), as well as astigmatism, are described by the dioptric power of the lens prescribed to correct the defect (resulting in descriptions like "the patient is a 4 diopter myope"); 3. measure of the refracting power of a prism; *see* prism diopter.

dioptric: Adjectival form of diopter.

diplopia: Perception of two images where there is only one object (colloquially known as *double vision*); *see also* multiple vision *and* polyopia; **binocular d.** double vision resulting from the lack of fusion of the images from each eye; **crossed d.** double vision in which the image from one eye is seen on the opposite side of the image from the fellow eye; **horizontal d.** doubled images are side-by-side; **monocular d.** double image seen with only one eye rather than both, resulting from some abnormality of the ocular media or a neurological problem in processing the image from the retina; **vertical d.** double vision in which the two images are one above the other.

direct illumination: In slit lamp biomicroscopy, method of viewing by shining light from the slit lamp upon the ocular structures to be viewed; *compare* indirect illumination.

direct ophthalmoscopy: Process of viewing a magnified image of the inside of the eye; it is called *direct* because the image is seen right-side-up; most often referring to the use of a hand-held ophthalmoscope through which the examiner looks with one eye (thus obtaining only a two-dimensional image with no depth); *compare* indirect ophthalmoscopy.

disciform keratitis: *See* keratitis.

disk (or, less preferred, disc) (d): General anatomic term for flat, circular structures; in ophthalmic usage, portion of the retina where nerve fibers converge to form the optic nerve (more properly called the *optic disk* or the *optic nerve head*).

disk drusen: *See* drusen.

dispensing: In ophthalmic usage, the business of selling spectacles and/or contact lenses; includes fitting, adjusting, and educating the customer.

dissociated vertical deviation (DVD): *See* deviation.

distance between centers (DBC): Distance, in millimeters, between the optical centers of lenses mounted in a pair of spectacles; usually equal to the patient's pupillary distance.

distance between lenses (DBL): Width of the bridge of a pair of spectacles at its narrowest point, in millimeters.

distance vision: Vision of objects relatively far from the eye, approaching infinity; the distance at which visual tasks such as driving are considered to be performed, generally defined to be a minimum of about 20 feet; *compare* near vision; *see also* vision.

distometer: Rotating conversion chart used to properly change lens power for varying vertex distances.

divergence: 1. In optics, the spreading outward of parallel light rays after passing through a minus lens; 2. outward turning of one or both eyes; *compare* convergence.

divergent lens: Another term for minus lens.

divergent strabismus: *See* strabismus.

Dk: Unit of measure of the oxygen transmission of contact lens materials, given as the product of the material's oxygen diffusion coefficient (D) times oxygen solubility (k) in the material at a given thickness, temperature, and hydration.

documentation: Permanent recording of the elements of a patient exam, including the history, the results of any tests, findings, proposed and recommended treatment, discussions with the patient, and other items; may be written, entered in a computer system, or tape recorded; may not be erased but may be corrected by further documentation; *see also* history.

doll's eye sign: Turning of the eyes in the opposite direction from which the head is moved; it is an attempt by the vestibular system to maintain fixation.

dominant eye: The eye that is subjectively preferred for use by an individual, much the way one hand or the other is preferred; *compare* nondominant eye.

Donders' law: In any tertiary (oblique) eye position, the extraocular muscles exert the same torsion, regardless of how the eye was moved to attain that direction of gaze.

Doppler ultrasound: Imaging technique in which the reflection of high-frequency sound waves from a moving object is analyzed to create a representation of the movement; used in ophthalmic applications to study ocular blood flow, especially in the retina.

dot-and-blot hemorrhage: Appearance of small hemorrhages in the tissues of the retina, usually associated with diabetic retinopathy but also seen with other conditions.

double concave lens: *See* concave lens.

double convex lens: *See* convex lens.

double vision: *See* diplopia.

drusen: Circular, yellowish bodies that appear on the choroid as a consequence of aging or in some retinal degenerations; vision is rarely affected.

dry eye syndrome: Common condition in which a defect in the composition or production of the tears or incomplete closure of the eyelids results in corneal dryness, discomfort, and possible risk to the cornea; *see also* keratoconjunctivitis sicca.

dry macular degeneration: *See* macular degeneration.

Duane's retraction syndrome: Abnormal function of the rectus muscles wherein the eye retracts into the orbit and the upper eyelid drops when the eye is moved in toward the nose.

duction: Movement of an eye by the extraocular muscles; *see also* forced duction test; *compare* vergence.

dye laser: *See* laser.

dynamic stabilization: Method of stabilizing toric contact lenses by thinning the upper and lower edges of the lens, which offers the least resistance to the lids during blinking and thus helps to prevent rotation and maintain the orientation of the lens to correct astigmatism in the proper axis; *compare* posterior toric, prism ballast, *and* truncation.

dyslexia: Impairment of reading ability not obviously attributable to any defect within the eye.

E

Eales' disease: Condition predominantly of young adult males characterized by repeated retinal hemorrhage.

eccentric fixation: State in which an eye fixates upon an object in such a way that the image of the object does not fall on the fovea, most often as compensation for damage in the area of the fovea.

ecchymosis: General medical term for discoloration due to hemorrhage within a tissue; bruising.

echography: Another term for ultrasonography.

ectatic corneal dystrophy: Another term for keratoconus.

ectopic: General medical term describing a dislocated organ, as in an ectopic lens or pupil.

ectropion: General medical term for the twisting inside-out of a structure, most commonly in ophthalmic usage referring to a condition in which the lid turns outward from the eye, exposing the conjunctiva; *compare* entropion.

edge glare: Unwanted scattering of light striking the edge of a contact lens or intraocular lens, perceived as streaks or other visual disturbances that reduce visual acuity.

edger: Machine used to trim lenses to fit into spectacle frames.

effective diameter (ED): The diagonal size of the eyewire (lens opening) in a pair of spectacles, measured in millimeters.

effective power: *See* back vertex power.

electroencephalography (EEG): Method of recording electric potentials in the brain.

electromagnetic spectrum: The range of energy waves conducted through the electrical fields present throughout space, from long-wavelength energy (eg, radio waves) to short-wavelength energy (eg, cosmic radiation); visible light includes the wavelengths from about 3800 to 7600 angstroms, recognized as colors from violet to red, respectively.

electro-oculography (EOG): Technique for analyzing the function of the retinal pigment epithelium via electrodes placed on the test subject's face; changes in electrical potential are recorded as the subject alternates the eyes from one fixation point to another.

electroretinography (ERG): Technique for measuring the response of the retina to light through electrodes placed on the surface of the globe.

elevator muscles: Extraocular muscles (ie, the superior rectus and inferior oblique) that move the eye upward.

Elschnig's pearls: Small whitish nodules of lens epithelium that sometimes appear on remnants of the lens capsule after cataract extraction.

Elschnig's spots: Small pale areas of dead choroidal tissue often associated with hypertension.

emmetrope: One who does not need corrective lenses to see well at near and far.

emmetropia: Condition in which the unaided eye properly focuses light onto the retina; *compare* ametropia.

emmetropization: Resolution of refractive error, usually referring to the resolution of hyperopia as a child grows.

encircling band: Another term for scleral buckle.

endocapsular: Appearing or occurring within the lens capsule; *see* phacoemulsification.

endolenticular: Appearing or occurring within the crystalline lens; *see* phacoemulsification.

endophthalmitis: Inflammation of the internal ocular tissues, occasionally an infection after surgery or penetrating injury that can lead to loss of vision and of the eye itself if not controlled; **bacterial e.** endophthalmitis caused by infection; **sterile e.** endophthalmitis caused by some agent other than infection.

endothelium: *See* corneal endothelium.

endpiece: Part on either side of a spectacle frame front to which the temples are attached.

enhancement: Euphemism for a repeat of treatment; the term has become well-established in ophthalmology, especially among refractive surgeons.

entropion: General term for an inward twisting of a structure, most commonly in ophthalmic usage a folding inward of the lid resulting in the lashes rubbing against the globe; *compare* ectropion.

enucleation: Removal of the whole eyeball after severing the muscle, nerve, and vascular attachments.

enucleation implant: Another term for orbital implant.

epicanthal fold: Fold of skin overlying the inner canthus, especially common and prominent in persons of Asian descent (sometimes called the *epicanthus*).

epidemic keratoconjunctivitis (EKC): *See* keratoconjunctivitis.

epikeratophakia: Epikeratoplasty performed as part of a cataract extraction procedure.

epikeratoplasty: Refractive surgical procedure in which donor corneal tissue is sutured over the patient's cornea (after removal of the corneal epithelium) to correct myopia, hyperopia, or astigmatism; somewhat unpredictable but reversible.

epinephrine: One of two biochemicals that conducts messages for the sympathetic nervous system (the other is norepinephrine); also called *adrenaline*; *see also* norepinephrine; *compare* acetylcholine.

epinucleus: Tissue surrounding the relatively harder crystalline lens nucleus.

epiphora: Excessive tear flow of the eyes due either to overproduction of tears or insufficient drainage by the lacrimal system.

epiretinal membrane (ERM): Detachment of the internal limiting membrane of the retina from the retina and vitreous body, occurring for a variety of reasons (eg, pathology, surgery, or trauma) and sometimes progressing to cellophane maculopathy (ie, wrinkling of the membrane) and macular pucker (ie, contraction of the membrane in the area of the macula).

episclera: Outermost layer of the sclera containing fine connective tissue and blood vessels.

epithelial ingrowth: Undesirable healing of corneal wounds or incisions in which the corneal epithelium invades the internal surfaces of the healing wound.

epithelial punctate keratitis: *See* keratitis.

epithelium: *See* corneal epithelium.

equator: General term for an imaginary line midway between two poles of a sphere; often used to describe the location of points on the eyeball or crystalline lens (eg, equatorial staphyloma or equatorial cataract).

error (refractive): Another term for ametropia.

erythrolabe: Visual pigment present in the "red" retinal cones that absorb light in the red frequencies (around 570 nm); one of three visual pigments; *see also* chlorolabe, cyanolabe, *and* trichromatism.

esodeviation: A deviation of the eyes in which one eye turns inward; may be latent (phoria) or manifest (tropia).

esophoria (E): Heterophoria in which one eye turns inward when deprived of the visual stimulus for fusion.

esotropia (ET): Type of strabismus in which one eye turns in toward the nose (also called *convergent deviation* or *convergent strabismus*); **A pattern e.** esotropia in which the eyes are more converged in up-gaze; **accommodative e.** esotropia usually appearing in the first few years of life in which excessive turning inward of the eye occurs during near vision; **acquired e.** esotropia that occurs after age one; **congenital (infantile) e.** large esotropia occurring in the first 6 months of life without significant refractive error; **intermittent e.** esotropia that is not present all the time (ie, the subject is sometimes able to fuse); **nonaccommodative e.** esotropia that measures the same even when fully corrected for hyperopia, including the latent component; *see also* hyperopia; **V pattern e.** esotropia in which the eyes are more converged in down-gaze.

ethmoid bone: One of the bones of the orbit.

ethylenediaminetetraacetic acid (EDTA): Preservative used in some fluid medications.

eversion: General medical term for a turning inside out; in ophthalmic practice, to evert the eyelid is to turn the lid inside out so the palpebral conjunctiva can be examined.

evisceration: Removal of the eyeball's contents.

evoked potential: *See* visual evoked potential.

excavation of optic disk: *See* cupping.

excimer laser: *See* laser.

exciter filter: Blue filter placed on the light source of the fundus camera to induce fluorescence of injected fluorescein dye for retinal photography and examination.

executive bifocal: Classic spectacle design in which the near (reading) segment of the lens extends across the entire width of the bottom of the lens with a clearly visible line dividing it from the upper far (distance) segment.

exenteration: Surgical removal of the globe in addition to orbital contents (eg, muscles, lids, etc).

exfoliation: General term for the process in which tissue flakes apart in scale-like pieces; while "true" exfoliation is considered to occur in the crystalline lens, in ophthalmic usage this term usually describes exfoliation/pseudoexfoliation syndrome, where flakes of ocular material appear on structures in the anterior chamber; *see also* pseudoexfoliation syndrome.

exodeviation: A deviation of the eyes in which one eye turns outward; may be latent (phoria) or manifest (tropia).

exophoria (X): Heterophoria in which an eye turns outward when deprived of a visual stimulus that stimulates fusion.

exophthalmia, -os: Protrusion of the eye(s); another term for proptosis.

exophthalmometer: Instrument used to measure eye protrusion.

exotropia (XT): Type of strabismus in which one eye is turned outward (also called *divergent deviation* or *divergent strabismus*); **A pattern e.** exotropia in which the deviation is greater in down-gaze; **constant e.** exotropia that is present all the time; **intermittent e.** exotropia that the subject can fuse (ie, hold the eyes straight) at some times and not others; **V pattern e.** exotropia in which the deviation is greater in up-gaze.

exposure keratitis: *See* keratitis.

expulsive hemorrhage: Sudden, heavy bleeding from the choroid and retina of the eye, most often occurring during a surgical procedure and having the potential to force ocular tissues out of the incision; it is the most dramatic and potentially most devastating intraoperative complication of ophthalmic surgery.

extended wear lens: Contact lens intended to be worn overnight or, in some cases, up to several weeks without removal; the cornea beneath the lens receives oxygen via the tears as well as through the lens material itself.

external limiting membrane (of retina): Zone of the retina intermingling with and directly under the photoreceptors (ie, rods and cones), forming the border with the outer nuclear layer.

external rectus muscle: Another name for lateral rectus muscle.

extort: To induce motion of an eye so that the "north pole" of the globe tilts outward away from the other eye; *compare* intort.

extracapsular cataract extraction: General term for surgical techniques in which the anterior lens capsule is partially or completely removed in order to facilitate cataract extraction, usually referring to procedures in which a lens loop is used to remove the lens as an intact unit; *see also* cataract extraction *and* phacoemulsification; *compare* intracapsular cataract extraction.

extraocular muscles (EOMs): Rectus and oblique muscles attached to the outside of the eye and the inside of the bony orbit; responsible for movements of the eyeball.

exudate: *See* retinal exudates.

exudative retinitis: *See* retinitis.

eye bank: Organization that serves as a clearing house for donated eyes, most importantly to provide corneas for penetrating keratoplasty but also to distribute eyes unsuitable for transplantation for use in research and training.

eye strain: Another term for asthenopia.

eyebrow: Row of hairs above the orbit at the brow, properly called *supercilium*.

eyelash: Fine, short hair arising from the margin of the eyelid; properly called *cilia*; plural: cilium.

eyelid: Either of two flaps of skin that cover the eye during blinking; *see also* combining forms beginning with blephar-, palpebr-, and tars-.

eyewire: Part of a spectacle frame front that holds the lens; each frame has a left and right eyewire joined by a bridge.

facultative hyperopia: *See* hyperopia.

facultative suppression: Mental "blocking out" of the image produced by one eye in order to prevent double vision, occurring only when the eye is deviated; *compare* obligatory suppression.

falciform fold: Fold of connective tissue where extraocular muscles attach to the globe.

far point of accommodation: *See* accommodation.

far point of convergence: *See* convergence.

Farnsworth test: Any one of several tests of color vision.

farsightedness: Another term for hyperopia.

fascia: General medical term for sheet of fibrous tissue covering an anatomic structure and providing it with attachment, support, and protection during movement.

fascia bulbi: Another term for Tenon's capsule.

FDA grid: Data from clinical studies of Food and Drug Administration-approved intraocular lenses compiled in the 1980s for evaluating future IOLs; it includes rates of sight-threatening complications as well as postoperative visual acuity.

fenestration: Practice of putting a tiny hole in a rigid contact lens in order to increase tear fluid exchange.

field: Another term for visual field.

field defect: *See* visual field defect.

field of view: The area in which one can see without turning the head or eyes.

filamentary keratitis: *See* keratitis.

filariasis: Parasitic infestation with threadworms, possibly affecting the eyes; *see also* onchocerciasis.

filtering bleb: *See* bleb *and* filtering operation.

filtering implant or **valve:** Device implanted to control intraocular pressure by allowing aqueous fluid to drain from the anterior chamber.

filtering operation: Surgical procedure used in treatment of glaucoma in which an opening is created through which aqueous fluid may pass from the anterior chamber into a sac (ie, bleb) created beneath the conjunctiva, thus lowering the pressure within the eye.

filtration angle: *See* angle.

finger counting vision: *See* count-finger vision.

fingerprint corneal dystrophy: *See* corneal dystrophy (map-dot-fingerprint).

fish-mouth: Undesirable postoperative condition in which the edges of a wound or incision fail to close but instead curl and gape open.

fitting triangle: Desirable method of adjusting and fitting spectacles so that the frames touch the patient *only* on the bridge of the nose and the top of each ear.

fixation: Also known as *central f.;* looking directly at an object so that its image falls on the macula; requires that the eyes be steady (*compare* nystagmus) and have a measure of visual function depending on the target; **binocular** or **bifoveal f.** ability to bring both eyes to bear upon the same object; requires coordination of ocular muscles; *see also* fusion; **eccentric f.** image does not fall on the macula but rather some peripheral retinal point, generally associated with long-standing amblyopia; **monocular f.** fixation of one eye (versus binocular f.).

fixation light or **target:** Device at which the patient looks to assist in maintaining fixation during an examination or treatment.

flap: In ophthalmic surgery, a piece of tissue dissected away from the eye but left attached at one edge so that it can be repositioned over the site of the operation.

flare: Presence of protein particles in the aqueous humor indicating intraocular inflammation, usually after surgery or trauma; *see also* cell.

flare and cell: In ophthalmic usage, usually the appearance of protein particles and white blood cells in the aqueous humor/anterior chamber, indicating intraocular inflammation.

flat: In ophthalmic usage, describing the surface curvature of a lens or ocular medium that imparts relatively low refractive power; *compare* steep.

flat axis: The least curved (and thus least refractive) of the principal meridians of a curved surface, either of the ocular media (cornea or lens) or a ground lens.

flat chamber: Collapse of the anterior chamber as a result of insufficient intraocular pressure, typically because of loss of aqueous humor due to trauma or surgical complication.

flat top spectacles: Bifocal spectacles in which the top of the bifocal segment is a straight line (as opposed to round).

flattening: In refractive surgery, decreasing the curvature of the cornea to correct myopia; *compare* steepening.

Fleischer ring: A brownish iron deposit in the corneal epithelium around the base of the cone in keratoconus.

flicker fusion test: Measure of retinal cone function in which the frequency of a flashing light is increased until the flashes are perceived as one continuous light.

Flieringa ring: Metal ring placed on the sclera during ophthalmic surgery to maintain the shape of the eye and prevent loss of vitreous humor.

floaters: Dark specks or strands in the field of view caused by cells or other nontransparent material in the vitreous.

flow: In ophthalmic surgery, the passing of irrigation fluid through the eye; *see also* aspiration flow rate.

fluence: In optics, the rate of delivery of light energy over time, usually used to describe the amount of laser energy being delivered to a treatment area.

fluid-gas exchange: Surgical procedure in which infusion fluid introduced into the posterior segment as part of retinal detachment repair is removed and replaced with air, a heavy synthetic gas, or a mixture of the two.

fluorescein: Yellowish fluorescent dye used in many ophthalmic diagnostic procedures; for examination of corneal surface defects it is used topically; for evaluation of the retinal vasculature it is injected intravenously.

fluorescein angiography (FA): Imaging technique in which fluorescein dye is injected into the arterial system; the dye fluoresces, revealing the circulatory system of the retina and choroid in vivo.

fluorescein clearance test: Assessment of the lacrimal system by applying fluorescein drops to the eye and timing how long it takes to drain away with the tear fluid.

fluorescein stain: Topical application of fluorescein to assess the condition of the corneal surface or the fit of a rigid contact lens.

fluorescence: Excitation of a material's electrons caused by light energy such that photons of light are emitted when the electrons fall back into their original orbits; this property is used in imaging techniques; *see* fluorescein angiography.

fluorophotometry: Method of assessing fluid flow (eg, the flow of aqueous humor through the anterior chamber) by measuring the concentration of fluorescein over time using a slit lamp fluorometer.

focal distance or **length:** Distance from a lens to the point at which rays of light converge to a focal point; if the power of a lens in diopters (D) is known, focal length in meters (F) is calculated using the formula $F = 1/D$.

focal point: The point at which the rays of light converge; *see also* image.

focus: 1. To bring together rays of light with an optical system so as to obtain an image of an object; 2. another term for *focal point*.

fogging: Purposely blurring vision by the addition of plus lenses either to eliminate accommodation (in refractometry) or to semiocclude the fogged eye.

foldable intraocular lens: *See* intraocular lens.

follicles: In ophthalmic usage, tiny clear or yellow sacs of lymphocytes and inflammatory cells appearing on the conjunctiva after prolonged irritation, often as a result of viral infection.

follicular conjunctivitis: *See* conjunctivitis.

foot-candle: Measure of the intensity of light falling on a given surface area, defined as one lumen per square foot.

foot lambert: Another term for foot-candle.

forced duction test: In ophthalmic usage, test in which an anesthetized eye is physically moved by the examiner to check for mechanical restrictions to movement; the ease with which the eye can be moved and the speed with which it returns to a neutral position are observed (also called *passive forced duction test*).

foreign body (FB): Any object lodged in ocular tissue, usually as a result of trauma; **inorganic f.b.** object from a nonliving source (such as metal); **organic f.b.** object from living source (such as plant or animal matter).

foreign body sensation: Perception that an object is lodged in ocular tissue, either because such an object (sometimes a postoperative suture) is actually present or because of an abrasion, inflammation, trichiasis, or other condition.

fornix: General medical term for an arch-like anatomic structure; in ophthalmic usage, the cul-de-sac (area where the bulbar conjunctiva folds over to become the palpebral conjunctiva).

fovea: Small depression in the center of the macula in which cone cells are densely packed; *see also* macula.

foveal avascular zone (FAZ): Central 0.3 to 0.45 mm area of the fovea in which there is no vascular supply.

foveola: Central pit of the fovea.

frame difference: The difference, in millimeters, between the horizontal (ie, "A" measurement) and vertical (ie, "B" measurement) measurement of the eyewires in a spectacle frame; has a bearing on lens thickness and position in that a thick lens has a better cosmetic appearance if the frame difference is small.

frame front: The two eyewires, bridge, and endpieces (where the temples are attached) of a pair of spectacles; *see also* temple.

frame pupillary distance (frame PD): Measurement, in millimeters, from the geometric (versus optical) center of the lenses in a pair of spectacles; taken by measuring from the nasal edge of one eyewire to the temporal edge of the other; also called the *geometric center distance* (GCD).

Fresnel lens: (pronounced fray-nell) lens composed of concentric rings that are sections of simple lenses of varying refractive power; it is thin yet provides great focusing or prismatic power although the optics are not as good as a regular lens.

front vertex power: Portion of the total refractive power imparted by the front surface of a lens; *compare* back vertex power.

frontal bone: One of the bones of the orbit.

Fuchs' dystrophy: The most common type of corneal endothelial dystrophy, characterized by the presence of guttata.

fundus: General term for the base of an organ or area (from the Latin for foundation); in ophthalmic usage, the retina, macula, optic disk, and retinal blood vessels as seen through an ophthalmoscope.

funduscopy: In ophthalmic usage, viewing the retinal fundus.

fusion: Binocular process in which each eye exerts the effort to fixate on the same object; **motor f.** action of the oculomotor system to align the eyes to achieve sensory fusion; **sensory f.** action of the brain in combining the slightly disparate images from each eye into one perceived, three-dimensional image; stereopsis cannot exist without fusion, but fusion can exist without stereopsis; *see also* stereopsis.

fusion amplitude: Range between the maximum convergence and maximum divergence that a test subject can tolerate while still maintaining fusion (ie, points at which fusion is lost); measured in prism diopters.

G

Galilean telescope: *See* telescope.

gamma angle: *See* angle.

ganglion: Cluster of nerve cell bodies.

ganglion cell layer: Retinal cell layer consisting of sensory cells whose axons form the fibers of the optic nerve.

gas-fluid exchange (GFE): Surgical procedure in which fluid introduced into the posterior segment as part of retinal detachment repair is removed and replaced with air, a heavy synthetic gas, or a mixture of the two.

gas-permeable contact lens (GPCL): *See* contact lens.

gaze: Reference to the direction in which one is fixating, especially in strabismus testing; **cardinal (diagnostic) positions of g.** eight directions of fixation that each exhibit the functions of various extraocular muscles; they are up, up and right, right, down and right, down, down and left, left, up and left; *see also* range of motion; **primary g.** position of fixating straight ahead.

Geneva lens measure: Another term for lens clock.

geniculate body: Area of the human brain that bridges the optic nerve and the cerebral cortex.

geometric center distance: Another term for frame pupillary distance.

giant papillary conjunctivitis (GPC): *See* conjunctivitis.

giant retinal break or **tear:** Retinal tear extending across three or more clock hours (90 degrees) of the eye.

glabella: Point immediately above the bridge of the nose between the eyebrows, used as a reference point, particularly in reconstructive and plastic surgery.

glare: Distortion in an optical system whereby light from point sources (eg, the sun or automobile headlights) is dispersed across the field of view; glare has been cited as a particular problem for cataract patients; *see also* glare test.

glare test: Test in which varying amounts of bright light are shown into the subject's eye during visual acuity evaluation; the purpose is to simulate room, outdoor, and full sun lighting; typically, visual acuity decreases in patients with cataracts (especially posterior subcapsular) when glare is added; one widely-used instrument is the Brightness Acuity Tester (BAT).

glaucoma: Group of ocular disorders in which damage to the optic nerve and visual field loss are usually associated with high intraocular pressure; a leading cause of blindness throughout the world, glaucoma causes irreversible vision loss but in its early stages has no symptoms; *see also* glaucoma suspect *and* ocular hypertension; **acute angle-closure g.** sudden rise in intraocular pressure caused by blockage of the angle of the anterior chamber, marked by painful onset and extremely high pressure; **angle-closure g.** (AGC) *see* closed-angle g.; **angle-recession g.** type of secondary glaucoma following ocular trauma that tears the ciliary body, resulting in scarring and diminished outflow of aqueous fluid; **aphakic g.** elevated intraocular pressure after removal of the crystalline lens of the eye; **chronic g.** high intraocular pressure that is sustained over a prolonged time without any critical sudden rises, may be of closed- or open-angle type; **closed-angle g.** normal drainage though the angle is blocked off and aqueous fluid rapidly builds up in the anterior chamber, creating high intraocular pressure and nerve damage; may be acute or chronic; **congenital g.** rare form of glaucoma that is present at birth; **hemolytic g.** glaucoma caused by blockage of the angle of the anterior chamber by blood cells; **iris-**

block g. glaucoma caused when the iris blocks the angle; **juvenile g.** glaucoma occurring in youth; **low-pressure** or **low-tension g.** glaucoma occurring at an intraocular pressure usually considered to be within the normal or low range; **malignant g.** postoperative elevation of intraocular pressure that occurs when the anterior chamber is flattened from behind (ie, the posterior segment's volume is increased), closing the angle; **neovascular g.** glaucoma caused by growth of blood vessels into the angle of the anterior chamber, which impairs outflow of aqueous fluid; **normal pressure g.** another term for low-pressure glaucoma; **open-angle g.** glaucoma caused by build-up of aqueous fluid in the anterior chamber due to impaired outflow through the tissue spaces of the angle even though the angle is open; **phacolytic g.** glaucoma resulting from leakage of lens proteins in very advanced cases of cataract; **pigmentary g.** glaucoma resulting from iris pigment dispersed into the angle; *compare* pigmentary dispersion syndrome in which no glaucoma occurs; **primary g.** general term for glaucoma unrelated to previous disease (generally divided into primary closed-angle and primary open-angle glaucoma); **pupillary block g.** glaucoma caused when the crystalline lens crowds against the iris, obstructing the pupil and trapping aqueous; **secondary g.** glaucoma resulting from disease or injury; may be open-angle or closed-angle; *compare* primary g.

glaucoma suspect: Situation in which the patient exhibits symptoms that indicate glaucoma may occur or already exists; *see also* ocular hypertension.

glaucomatous: Like or of glaucoma.

glaucomatous cataract: Opacification caused by high intraocular pressure.

glaucomatous cupping: *See* cupping.

globe: Another term for the eyeball.

goblet cells: Mucin-producing cells found in mucus membranes; in the eye, goblet cells are located in the conjunctiva and produce the mucin found in tears.

Goldmann applanation tonometer: *See* tonometer.

Goldmann lens: *See* goniolens.

Goldmann perimeter: *See* perimetry.

Goldmann tonometer: *See* tonometer.

goniolens: Lens, typically incorporating several mirrors, that allows one to see or direct laser energy into the angle of the anterior chamber; the lens is placed directly onto the anesthetized eye; many configurations are available, including the Goldmann, Hruby, Karickhoff, Koeppe, and Zeiss lenses.

goniophotocoagulation: Laser procedure for treatment of glaucoma that attempts to lower intraocular pressure by using laser energy (directed by a goniolens) to open the trabecular meshwork; *see* trabeculectomy.

gonioscopy: Examination of the angle of the anterior chamber using a goniolens.

grade I, II, III, and IV: Many medical conditions, including ophthalmic entities such as capsular opacification, cataract, corneal haze, etc, are assessed by assigning subjective grades from I (or 1, noticeable) to IV (or 4, severe); although some researchers periodically attempt to define objective criteria for the grades assigned to these various conditions, clinicians prefer to establish their own definitions for use in patient records; *see* Appendix 7.

gram stain: Dye used to classify bacteria; gram-positive bacteria stain dark blue and gram-negative bacteria stain red.

Graves' disease: Thyroid overactivity generally resulting in exophthalmos but sometimes also associated with dysfunction of extraocular muscle and optic nerve as well as corneal involvement; ocular involvement is also called *thyroid eye disease*.

grid: *See* Amsler grid *or* FDA grid.

Gullstrand's schematic/reduced eye: *See* schematic eye, definition 2.

Gunn's pupil: *See* Marcus Gunn pupil.

guttata: General medical colloquialism for a spot or spots with the appearance of water droplets; in ophthalmic usage, referring to the appearance of such spots on the inner surface of the cornea; *see* endothelial corneal dystrophy *under* corneal dystrophy; plural: indeterminable, although guttata as the singular and guttatae as the plural seem to be well accepted.

H

half-glasses: Spectacles that have only the lower half of a lens, used to provide correction for near vision to presbyopes who find their uncorrected distance vision acceptable.

halo: Distortion in an optical system that causes rings to be seen around point sources of light.

hand-motion vision (HM): Very low level of visual acuity in which no greater detail can be perceived other than the motion of a hand waved before the eyes; *see also* count-finger vision, light perception vision, no light perception vision, *and* visual acuity.

haploscope: Instrument that presents two separate fields of view to the two eyes for evaluation of binocular vision.

haptic: Portion of an intraocular lens comprised of a thin arm that curves outward from the optic, sometimes referred to as a *loop*.

hard exudates: *See* retinal exudates.

harmonious retinal correspondence (HRC): State in which corresponding points from the two images focused on each retina are properly associated in the image created by fusion in the brain; also called *normal retinal correspondence (NRC)*; *compare* anomalous retinal correspondence.

haze: General term in ophthalmic usage for cloudiness of normally clear optical medium, usually referring to the cornea.

heavy fluid or **gas:** Any of several materials used in posterior segment surgery to replace the vitreous humor following vitrectomy, often as part of retinal detachment repair; these materials include perfluorocarbons such as perfluoropropane (C_3F_8), silicone oil, and sulfur hexafluoride (SF_6).

HEMA: Hydroxyethylmethacrylate, polymer from which most soft hydrogel contact lenses are made; *see* hydrogel.

hemianopia, -opsia: Partial or total loss of vision in half the visual field in one or both eyes; the upper or lower portions of the visual field, as well as the right and left sides, can be affected; **absolute h.** total loss of all visual perception in half the visual field; **altitudinal h.** loss of the upper or lower half of the visual field; **bilateral h.** partial or total loss of vision affecting the visual field of both eyes (also called *true hemianopia*); **binocular h.** another term for bilateral hemianopia; **binasal h.** loss of the half of the visual field on the side nearest the nose in each eye (ie, left field of the right eye and right field of the left eye); **bitemporal h.** loss of the temporal field in each eye (ie, right field in the right eye, left field of the left eye); **homonymous h.** loss of half the field in both eyes such that the loss is the same (superimposable) in each eye; **incongruous h.** loss of half the field in both eyes such that the loss is not identical in each eye; **quadrant h.** loss of one quarter of the visual field in each eye (also called a *quadrantanopia*); **unilateral h.** loss of half the visual field of only one eye.

HeNe laser: *See* laser, helium-neon.

Henle's fibers: Nerve fibers that join the rod and cone cells of the retina in the area of the fovea.

Hering's law of simultaneous innervation: Physiologic principle that the nerve stimulus generated by the oculomotor system to move the fixating eye is duplicated for the yoke muscle of the other eye, resulting in parallel movement of the eyes; *see also* yoke muscle.

Herpes zoster ophthalmicus: Herpetic viral infection affecting the trigeminal nerve (CN V) and the eye, generally as a part of shingles (which can occur without ocular involvement).

hetero-: Prefix meaning *different*.

heterochromia: General anatomic term describing a tissue or organ that shows a mottling of colors when normally it is of a single hue (eg, a heterochromic iris); *compare* isochromatic.

heteronymous diplopia: Double vision in which the image seen by the right eye is perceived to be to the left of the image seen by the left eye; also known as *crossed diplopia; compare* homonymous diplopia.

heterophoria: Another term for phoria.

heterophthalmia: General term for the difference in structure or function between the two eyes.

heteropsia: State in which one eye has different visual characteristics (eg, degree of myopia) than the fellow eye.

heterotropia: Another term for tropia.

hippus: Rhythmic contraction and dilation of the pupils independent of any stimulus, often seen when shining a light into the eye in order to evaluate pupillary reflexes; not usually indicative of pathology.

Hirschberg's test: Identification of tropia by noting the position of the reflections of a fixation light on the patient's corneas; if both reflections are on the visual axis (slightly nasal), the eyes are orthotropic, but if the reflection is on axis in one eye but not the other, a tropia may be present.

history: Process of interviewing the patient in order to document his or her medical conditions, past and present, both systemic and ocular; includes family history, social history, medications, allergies, signs, symptoms, aggravating and relieving factors, as well as answers to pertinent questions regarding the patient's complaint(s); *see also* documentation.

HIV: *See* human immunodeficiency virus.

homogenous keratoplasty: Keratoplasty in which the tissue comes from a donor (of the same species); *compare* autogenous keratoplasty.

homonymous diplopia: Double vision in which the image seen by the right eye is perceived to be to the right of the image seen by the left eye; also known as *uncrossed diplopia; compare* heteronymous diplopia.

homonymous field defect: Visual field defect that is the same in each eye (eg, both left halves of each visual field); *compare* incongruous field defect.

Honan balloon: Device placed on the eye before ophthalmic surgery designed to put pressure on the eye in order to reduce intraocular pressure.

hordeolum: Infection of one of the glands on the edge of the eyelid (**external h.** or sty) or in the palpebral conjunctiva (**internal h.**); *see also* meibomian cyst; *compare* chalazion.

horizontal prism bar: *See* prism bar.

Horner's syndrome: Disorder of the third cranial nerve causing miosis, ptosis, and anhidrosis (lack of sweating) on the affected side.

horopter: An imaginary arc that allows correlation of points in space to points on the retina; images in front of or behind the horopter will be perceived as double; *see also* Panum's fusion area.

horseshoe tear: Retinal tear in which a U-shaped flap of retinal tissue (attached on one side) is pulled away from the retina.

HOTV test: Visual acuity test for children in which the letters H, O, T, and V on a chart are matched to the same letters on cards.

Hruby contact lens: *See* goniolens.

human immunodeficiency virus (HIV): Virus implicated in acquired immunodeficiency syndrome (AIDS).

humor: General term for a fluid; **aqueous h.** *see* aqueous fluid; **vitreous h.** *see* vitreous body.

hyaloid membrane: In ophthalmic usage, the thin membrane that surrounds the vitreous, consisting of anterior hyaloid membrane (also called the *vitreous face*) and posterior hyaloid membrane.

hyaluronic acid: Component of certain viscoelastic substances.

hydrodelamination or **hydrodelineation:** In ophthalmic usage, surgical technique in which fluid is injected into the lens nucleus in order to break it up to facilitate cataract extraction.

hydrodissection: Most often in ophthalmic usage, surgical technique in which water is injected between tissue layers in order to separate them, usually employed in cataract extraction to separate the lens nucleus from the surrounding cortex; *compare* viscodissection.

hydrogel: Material used to make contact lenses and intraocular lenses; the hydrogel polymer (centered around the hydroxyethylmethacrylate [HEMA] molecule) is hydrophilic, which means that it can absorb large amounts of water and theoretically is more "friendly" to living tissue than hydrophobic materials.

hydrophilic: Describing a material that readily absorbs water.

hydrophobic: Describing a material that repels water.

hydrops: General medical term for accumulation of watery fluid in tissue; **corneal h.** aqueous fluid accumulation within the cornea due to decreased tissue integrity of the corneal endothelium and Descemet's membrane.

hydroxyethylmethacrylate (HEMA): *See* hydrogel.

hypermature cataract: *See* cataract.

hypermetropia: Another term for hyperopia.

hyperope: Individual with hyperopia.

hyperopia: Visual defect in which the eye focuses rays of light so that the focal point is behind the retina; commonly known as *farsightedness*, the hyperopic eye is not able to see objects that are nearby; **absolute h.** farsightedness that cannot be compensated for by accommodation; measured as the least amount of plus needed to produce clear vision; **axial h.** farsightedness attributable to the length of the eye (ie, the eye is too short for the refractive power of the cornea and crystalline lens); **facultative h.** another term for *manifest h.*; **latent h.** farsightedness that can be overcome by accommodation, generally measurable only during cycloplegia; **manifest h.** the amount of farsightedness that falls between absolute and latent hyperopia; figured as the difference between the measurement for absolute hyperopia and the maximum amount of plus the noncyclopleged patient can accept and still retain clear vision; **refractive h.** farsightedness that is attributable to the refractive power of the eye (ie, the cornea and lens are too weak to bring the incoming rays of light to focus on the retina).

hyperopic keratomileusis: *See* keratomileusis.

hyperosmotics: Class of drugs that reduce intraocular pressure by drawing aqueous out of the eye, most commonly used to treat acute angle-closure glaucoma (eg, glycerin, isosorbide, mannitol).

hyperphoria: Phoria in which one eye drifts upward when fusion is broken (generally by occluding the eye).

hypertelorism: General medical term for an abnormally large distance between two anatomic structures; in ophthalmic usage, an abnormally large distance between the eyes, a congenital condition usually accompanied by problems with ocular alignment and motility.

hypertropia: Strabismus in which the nonfixating eye turns upward relative to the fixating eye.

hyphema: Bleeding into the anterior chamber of the eye.

hypophoria: Phoria in which one eye drifts downward when fusion is broken (generally by occluding the eye).

hypopyon: Collection of pus in the anterior chamber of the eye.

hypotelorism: General medical term for an abnormally small distance between two anatomic structures; in ophthalmic usage, an abnormally small distance between the eyes.

hypotony: In ophthalmic usage, abnormally low intraocular pressure; *see also* intraocular pressure.

hypotropia: Strabismus in which the nonfixating eye turns downward relative to the fixating eye.

hypoxia: Abnormal reduction in the amount of oxygen available to a tissue; in ophthalmic usage, most frequently referring to lack of oxygen to the cornea related to contact lens wear; also called *anoxia* or *oxygen deprivation*.

hysterical: General medical term for a disorder triggered by emotional struggles; in ophthalmic usage, visual disorders due to emotional rather than organic causes; **h. blindness** *see* blindness; **h. visual field** *see* visual field defect.

I

illiterate E: Vision test target used for subjects who cannot read; the letter E is arranged in different directions, with rows of graded sizes, and the subject indicates which direction the "fork" of the letter E is pointing (of the smallest size E that is seen).

image: The representation of an object that is produced at the focal point of an optical system; **real i.** image produced at the focal point of a plus lens; this image is formed behind the lens and can thus be projected onto a screen; **virtual i.** image produced at the focal point of a minus lens, which, because it is formed in front of the lens, can only be stipulated to exist.

implant: General term for man-made material designed for surgical insertion into the human body; *see also* filtering implant, intraocular lens, *and* orbital implant.

incident light: Ray of light that enters a medium; *see also* reflection *and* refraction.

inclusion bodies or **inclusions:** General medical term for foreign particles seen within cells or tissues where they do not belong; in ophthalmic usage, often referring to particles of an unknown nature seen in the cornea.

inclusion conjunctivitis: *See* conjunctivitis.

incomitant (strabismus): *See* strabismus.

incongruous: General term indicating dissimilarity in form.

incongruous field defect: Visual field defects in both eyes that do not match each other; *compare* homonymous field defect.

index of refraction (IR): *See* refractive index.

indirect illumination: In slit lamp biomicroscopy, method of viewing an ocular structure by reflected light in which the slit lamp light is directed onto some other ocular structure than the one to be viewed; *see also* retroillumination; *compare* direct illumination.

indirect lens: A hand-held lens used during indirect ophthalmoscopy.

indirect ophthalmoscopy: Process of viewing the inside of the eye through instrumentation consisting of a light source and lens/prism viewer worn on the examiner's head and a loose lens held in front of the patient's eye; called *indirect* because the image is seen upside-down and reversed; because the examiner uses both eyes, however, the image is three-dimensional; *compare* direct ophthalmoscopy.

indocyanine green (ICG): Dye used in ophthalmology to image the choroid.

induced: 1. In ophthalmic surgical usage, usually referring to a condition that is a result (often unwanted) of surgery, such as induced astigmatism following cataract surgery; another term for *consecutive*; 2. in optics, the prismatic effect that occurs when the optical centers of a lens do not coincide with the patient's optical axis; *see* prism.

infantile: General medical term describing a feature or process (eg, glaucoma or cataract) that occurs during the first 2 years of life; *compare* congenital, juvenile, and senile.

inferior oblique (IO) muscle: Extraocular muscle lying underneath the eye around the equator of the globe responsible for elevating, abducting, and extorting the eye.

inferior rectus (IR) muscle: Extraocular muscle lying underneath the eye responsible for adducting, depressing, and extorting the eye.

infiltrates: Small particles that appear in tissue that is normally free of such particles; **corneal i.** whitish, cloudy particles in the cornea, often associated with infection or contact lens wear; **sterile i.** infiltrates, usually of the cornea, that are not associated with infection.

infiltrative keratitis: *See* keratitis.

infinity: In optics, imaginary point at distance from which rays of light travel in parallel paths; in clinical settings, 20 feet or more is considered to be infinity (thus, the denominator 20 for distance acuity measured using the Snellen's test chart).

informed consent: Process of explaining a treatment or procedure to the patient prior to its implementation, including risks and benefits such that the patient can sign a legal form stating that he or she understands the information presented; no surgery should ever be performed without prior informed consent by the patient or the patient's guardian.

infraorbital: At the bottom of or beneath the bony eye socket.

infusion: The act of introducing fluid into a closed anatomic structure, usually during surgery, or the fluid itself; *see also* irrigation.

injection: 1. The act of introducing fluid into tissue through a needle; 2. condition in which tissue is red, swollen, and engorged with dilated blood vessels; most often in ophthalmic usage referring to conjunctival injection.

inner molecular layer (of retina): Cell layer within the retina composed primarily of nerve synapses and containing the amacrine cells, located between the ganglion cell layer and the inner nuclear layer; also called the *inner granular layer*; *see also* retina.

inner nuclear layer (of retina): Cell layer within the retina composed primarily of bipolar cells and containing the capillaries that supply blood to the retina, located between the inner and outer molecular layers; *see also* retina.

insufficiency: *See* accommodative insufficiency *and* convergence insufficiency.

interferometer: Instrument that measures visual acuity by using a laser to project a target onto the retina, bypassing the ocular media (and any opacities therein); the target is a grating, which is adjustable to decrease in size and spacing; the results indicate what the patient's probable vision would be if any media opacities were removed; *see also* potential acuity meter.

intermittent: Not present at all times; in ophthalmology, often referring to strabismus; *see also* definitions for esotropia, exotropia, and strabismus.

internal limiting membrane (of the retina) (ILM): Innermost layer of the retina, in direct contact with the vitreous humor; also called the *hyaloid face of the vitreous*; *see also* retina.

internal rectus muscle: Another term for medial rectus muscle.

interpupillary distance (IPD): *See* pupillary distance.

intort: To induce motion of an eye so that the "north pole" (ie, 12 o'clock position) of the globe tilts inward toward the other eye (ie, clockwise for the right eye and counterclockwise in the left); *compare* extort.

intracameral: General medical term describing an entity located or occurring within a chamber; in ophthalmic usage, either within the anterior or posterior chamber.

intracameral anesthesia: Anesthetic agent injected into the anterior chamber of the eye, usually during cataract surgery.

intracapsular cataract extraction (ICCE): General term for surgical techniques in which cataract extraction is accomplished either by grasping the lens (within its intact capsule) with forceps or cryoextraction; ICCE has been almost completely abandoned (except in economically underdeveloped areas of the world) in favor of extracapsular procedures; *see also* cataract extraction; *compare* extracapsular cataract extraction.

intracapsular ligament: Connective tissue joining the extraocular muscles to the globe.

intracorneal: Within the cornea.

intracorneal implant: *See* intrastromal corneal ring.

intraocular: General anatomic term for structure, entity, or process appearing or occurring within the eye.

intraocular lens (IOL): Artificial lens surgically implanted into the eye to correct a refractive error, especially after cataract extraction; the age of contemporary intraocular lenses is considered to have begun in 1949 with the first implantation of an IOL made of polymethylmethacrylate; contemporary IOLs are manufactured in many designs from a variety of materials, but all have in common a central focusing portion (the optic) and supporting structures (the haptics); **acrylic IOL** foldable IOL manufactured from a polymer containing acrylic materials; **anterior chamber IOL** or **lens (ACL or A/C IOL)** IOL designed to be implanted in front of the iris, either after cataract extraction to correct aphakia or with the crystalline lens still in place to correct a refractive error; *compare* posterior chamber IOL; **C-loop IOL** IOL whose haptics are shaped like the letter C; **disk IOL** IOL with one circular haptic, designed to be implanted in the lens capsule to achieve centration; **foldable IOL** lens implant that can be folded, by virtue of either lens design or choice of soft lens material, and inserted into the eye through a small incision; **hydrogel IOL** foldable IOL manufactured from a polymer based upon the hydroxyethylmethacrylate (HEMA) molecule; **J-loop IOL** IOL whose haptics are shaped like the letter J; **phakic IOL** lens implanted to improve visual acuity while the natural crystalline lens remains in place; **piggyback IOLs** two IOLs implanted in the same eye in order to provide higher refractive correction than is possible with a single IOL; **plate-haptic IOL** IOL designed with flat, more or less solid plates instead of "arms" for haptics; **posterior chamber IOL** or **lens (PCL)** IOL designed to be implanted behind the iris, in either the lens capsule ("in the bag") or in the ciliary sulcus; *compare* anterior chamber IOL; **secondary IOL (2° IOL)** IOL implanted in a separate procedure some time after the crystalline lens has been removed; **silicone IOL** foldable IOL manufactured from a polymer based upon the silicone molecule; **soft IOL** *see* foldable IOL.

intraocular lens exchange: Surgical procedure to remove one IOL and replace it with another, either to replace a damaged or dislocated IOL or to insert the appropriate power lens if the first lens failed to correct vision sufficiently.

intraocular pressure (IOP): Pressure within the eye caused by the dynamics of the formation and drainage of aqueous humor; measured like atmospheric pressure as the height of a column of mercury that the pressure can support, thus the unit of measure is millimeters of mercury (mmHg); *see also* glaucoma, hypotony, *and* ocular hypertension.

intraorbital: Within the bony eye socket.

intraorbital implant: Device, usually composed of a bone-like substance, implanted in the orbit after the eye is removed due to disease; often designed to accept a prosthetic eye.

intrastromal: General medical term for location within the main substance of a tissue; in ophthalmic usage, referring to the corneal stroma.

intrastromal corneal ring: Device, shaped like a lens, ring, or portion of a ring, implanted within the cornea to correct a refractive error.

intravitreal: Located within the vitreous humor.

intumescent cataract: *See* cataract.

irid-: Root word meaning iris.

iridectomy: Surgical procedure to remove iris tissue to facilitate the flow of aqueous humor and thus lower or prevent a rise in intraocular pressure; *compare* iridotomy; **peripheral i. (PI)** removal of a small wedge of iris tissue near its edge (ie, away from the pupil); **sector i.** iridectomy in which a portion of the iris from the edge of the pupil to the outer edge of the iris is removed (resulting in a keyhole pupil); **total i.** *see* sector i.

iridemia: Bleeding from the iris.

irides: Plural of iris.

iridocorneal angle: *See* angle, definition 2.

iridocorneal endothelial syndrome: Condition in which corneal and iris endothelial cells proliferate, causing adhesions between the iris and cornea as well as blocking the iridocorneal angle, resulting in intraocular pressure rise.

iridocyclitis: Inflammation of the iris and ciliary body.

iridodialysis: Detachment of the root of the iris from the ciliary body.

iridodonesis: Abnormal anteroposterior movement ("flopping") of the iris, most often seen in aphakia or other situations in which the crystalline lens is displaced.

iridoplegia: Partial or total paralysis of the iris.

iridotomy: Surgical procedure to create an opening in the iris to provide a drainage point for aqueous, and prevent build-up of intraocular pressure; *see also* laser iridotomy; *compare* iridectomy.

iris: Mobile, vascular, ring-shaped structure that lies behind the cornea and in front of the crystalline lens; its movements control the size of the pupil and, thus, the amount of light passing through to the retina; attached at its outer edge to the ciliary body and covered with a (usually) highly pigmented epithelial layer; the pupillary zone of the iris contains the iris sphincter (sphincter pupillae), which constricts the pupil, and the ciliary zone contains the outer dilator muscle (dilator pupillae), which dilates the pupil; the collarette is the border between the sphincter and dilator; the iris divides the anterior and posterior chambers of the eye, although surgical procedures involving the lens and ciliary body, both of which lie behind the iris, are described as anterior segment surgery; plural: irides.

iris-block glaucoma: *See* glaucoma.

iris bombé: "Ballooning" of the iris outward into the anterior chamber caused by a build-up of fluid behind the iris; *see also* pupillary block.

iris coloboma: *See* coloboma.

iris crypts: Normally occurring furrows in the front surface of the iris.

iris hooks: Surgical instruments used to catch the edge of the iris in order to pull and hold open the pupil during surgery.

iris nevus: Small benign area, either smooth or slightly elevated, of excess pigment on the iris.

iris prolapse: Protrusion of part of the iris through a wound or surgical incision.

iris root: Area of the iris where it inserts into the ciliary body.

iris sphincter: Circular muscle within the iris surrounding the pupil and responsible for constriction of the pupil.

iritis: Inflammation of the iris characterized by pain, photophobia, and redness.

iron lines: Brown to black lines in the cornea caused by iron deposits.

irregular astigmatism: *See* astigmatism.

irrigation: General surgical term for washing a surface or cavity with fluid; *see also* infusion.

irrigation and aspiration (I&A, IA, or I/A): Surgical instrument and technique for removing intraocular tissue by simultaneously injecting fluid (ie, irrigation) and applying suction (ie, aspiration).

ischemic optic neuropathy (ION): Damage to the optic nerve because of obstructed blood flow, usually resulting in sudden blindness with a poor prognosis for recovery.

iseikonia: Normal condition in which each eye receives an image of similar size; *compare* aniseikonia.

Ishihara's test: Test for red/green color deficiency.

isochromatic: Uniformity of color, either between two or more objects or between different parts of the same object (as in an iris that is of a uniform color); *compare* anisochromatic.

isocoria: Normal condition in which the pupils of the two eyes are the same size; *compare* anisocoria.

isometropia: State in which both eyes have basically the same refractive power; *compare* anisometropia.

isopter: General term for line on a chart or map connecting similar numerical values; in ophthalmic usage, lines on a visual field test chart connecting the border of an area that responds to the same test object.

J

J-loop lens: *See* intraocular lens.

Jackson cross cylinder lens: *See* cross cylinder.

Jaeger's acuity (J): Measurement of visual acuity at near distances (reading acuity) based upon standard sizes of printed block letters, recorded as J1, J2, etc.

juvenile: Describing a feature or process (eg, cataract or glaucoma) appearing or occurring in late childhood; *compare* congenital, infantile, *and* senile.

K-reading: Usually referring to corneal curvature as measured during keratometry, less often referring to measurement of corneal thickness; *see* pachymetry.

kappa angle: *See* angle.

Karickhoff lens: *See* goniolens.

Kelman phacoemulsification: *See* phacoemulsification.

kerat-, -o-: Root word meaning literally horn, usually referring to the cornea but also describing other "hard" tissues such as fingernails.

keratectomy: General term for surgical removal of corneal tissue, usually performed as part of a corneal graft procedure; *see* keratoplasty; also, excimer laser surgery is described as photorefractive keratectomy because wide areas of corneal tissue are removed.

keratic precipitates (KPs): Small white or yellow bodies composed of inflammatory cells that adhere to the corneal endothelium, usually in the lower portion of the anterior chamber, seen in cases of iritis and iridocyclitis; **granulomatous** or **mutton-fat k.p.** large keratic precipitates resulting from long-standing inflammatory conditions; **punctate k.p.** small keratic precipitates.

keratitis: General term for inflammation of the cornea; *Acanthamoeba* **k.** inflammation of the cornea resulting from an infection with the *Acanthamoeba* organism, almost always associated with contact lens wear; **annular k.** inflammation and appearance of deposits around the periphery of the cornea; **bacterial k.** corneal inflammation caused by a nonviral infection; **band k.** *see* keratopathy; **dendriform** or **dendritic k.** branched lesion appearing on the cornea in Herpes virus infections; **disciform k.** disk-shaped edema deep in corneal tissue, often as a result of previous viral infection or inflammation; **epithelial punctate k.** *see* superficial punctate k.; **exposure k.** condition of corneal dryness, usually resulting from deficiency of tear fluid and/or incomplete closure of the eyelids during sleep; **filamentary k.** appearance of filaments attached to the corneal epithelium, can be a result of many conditions such as dry eye, infection, corneal abrasion, etc; **Herpes** or **Herpetic k.** Herpes virus infection leading to inflammation and lesions that may progress to ulcers; **infiltrative k.** corneal inflammation associated with whitish, cloudy particles, often indicating an infection or sometimes as a result of contact lens wear; **lattice k.** another term for lattice dystrophy; *see* corneal dystrophy; **punctate k.** condition in which infiltrates form in tiny points on the corneal endothelium, usually associated with viral infection; **superficial punctate k. (SPK)** condition in which elevated opacities (which stain when fluorescein is used) form in small points on the surface of the corneal epithelium, usually centrally; **viral k.** corneal inflammation caused by a viral infection.

keratitis sicca: *See* keratoconjunctivitis sicca.

keratoconjunctivitis: Inflammation of the tiss\[cornea and conjunctiva simultaneously; **atopic k.** keratoconjunctivitis associated with unusual sensitivity to allergens; **epidemic k. (EKC)** viral conjunctivitis that is highly contagious; duration is up to 3 to 4 weeks; **phlyctenular k.** inflammation of the cornea and conjunctiva associated with the appearance of small blisters on both tissues; *see also* phlyctenule.

keratoconjunctivitis sicca (KCS): Condition in which there is dryness, redness, and itching of the cornea and conjunctiva, often associated with chronic insufficient tear production; *see also* dry eye syndrome.

keratoconus (KC): Progressive malformation of the cornea such that it is thin and cone-like in shape rather than rounded; causes painless visual distortion (due to astigmatism) and loss; also called *ectatic corneal dystrophy.*

keratoglobus: Malformation of the cornea such that it enlarges and protrudes in a globe-like shape, often with associated myopia and astigmatism.

keratomalacia: Progressive degeneration of the cornea as a result of vitamin A deficiency.

keratome: Surgical instrument used to cut the cornea, either to create an incision into the eye for cataract surgery or to slice across the cornea to create a button for transplantation or flap for refractive surgery; *see also* keratomileusis *and* keratoplasty.

keratometer: Any of several types of instrument used to measure the curvature of the cornea; the term usually refers to an instrument that measures the central 1.5 mm of the cornea, as long as the meridians of curvature are 90 degrees from each other; used in fitting contact lenses and intraocular lens selection; *see also* corneal topography.

keratometry: General term for measurement of the cornea, usually of corneal curvature (*see* keratometer) but sometimes referring to corneal thickness (*see* pachymetry).

keratomileusis: Any of several refractive surgical procedures in which a keratome is used to remove and/or
reshape corneal tissue to correct a refractive error;
automated lamellar k. (ALK) *see* entry under keratoplasty; **Barraquer's k.** procedure no longer in use in
which corneal tissue was removed, frozen, reshaped,
thawed, and replaced on the eye; **hyperopic k.** keratomileusis performed to correct farsightedness; **laser
epithelial k. (LASEK)** keratomileusis in which the
corneal epithelium is loosened and pushed away from
the central cornea, excimer laser ablation is applied,
then the epithelium is replaced; **laser in-situ k.
(LASIK)** keratomileusis in which a keratome is used
to remove an outer layer of corneal tissue, a laser is
used to reshape the exposed corneal tissue, and then
the outer layer of corneal tissue is replaced (this technique is usually written and spoken as its abbreviation: LASIK); **myopic k.** keratomileusis performed to
correct nearsightedness.

keratopathy: General term for unhealthy condition of the
cornea; *see also* keratitis; **band k.** condition, usually
resulting from some underlying ocular or systemic
disease, marked by calcium deposits in Bowman's
layer which, as the name implies, appear across the
cornea in narrow bands; **bullous k.** degenerative condition of the cornea in which the epithelial cells form
small blisters (ie, bullae) that eventually burst; usually the result of some previous ocular disease;
pseudophakic bullous k. degenerative condition of
the cornea resulting from improper intraocular lens
implantation in which the endothelial cells form bullae; **ribbon k.** *see* band k.

keratophakia: Refractive surgical procedure in which a
thin slice of cornea is removed then replaced over a
suitably shaped piece of donor cornea (called a *lenticle*).

keratoplasty: General term for corneal grafting procedure (commonly called a *corneal transplant* or *corneal graft*) in which a patient's cornea is removed with a keratome and replaced with donor tissue (as is commonly done in cases of corneal disease) or after being reshaped (as is done in some refractive surgical procedures); **automated lamellar k. (ALK** or **AK)** procedure in which a keratome is used first to remove an outer layer of corneal tissue and then to remove an inner layer of tissue; the outer layer of tissue is then replaced on the eye, the shape of the removed inner layer determines the change in the eye's refractive state; **lamellar k. (LK** or **LKP)** surgical procedure to treat corneal opacity by removing the layer of corneal tissue in the area of the opacity and replacing it with a clear corneal graft; also called *partial penetrating k.*; **penetrating k. (PKP)** surgical procedure to treat corneal opacity in which the entire depth of a section of cornea is removed and replaced by a graft; also called *full-thickness k.*; **refractive k.** general term for keratoplasty performed to correct a refractive error.

keratoprosthesis: Artificial device used to replace the cornea either permanently in an attempt to restore sight (rarely used and rarely successful) or temporarily to facilitate some other operative procedure prior to replacing the cornea with a graft.

keratorefractive surgery: *See* refractive surgery.

keratoscopy: Technique for measuring the shape of the cornea by projecting evenly spaced, concentric circles of light (ie, keratometric mires) onto it; irregularities of the shape of the circles or the width of the space between them show deviations from a perfectly spherical shape; *see also* Placido's disk.

keratotomy: Surgical procedure in which incisions are made into the cornea; usually referring to refractive surgical procedures in which incisions are carefully placed in the cornea so that the natural healing response and structural changes that ensue will reshape the cornea and correct any refractive errors present; **arcuate** or **astigmatic k. (AK)** keratotomy consisting of curved incisions (with the arc centered on the optical axis) performed to correct astigmatism; **radial k. (RK)** refractive surgical procedure in which corneal incisions are placed radially, like the spokes of a wheel (leaving a central optical zone free of incisions), in order to flatten the cornea and correct near-sightedness; the degree of flattening depends upon the depth (about 90% of the corneal thickness) and number (typically from four to eight) of incisions.

keyhole pupil: Condition in which the pupil resembles a keyhole following a sector iridectomy.

kinetic perimetry: *See* perimetry.

Koeppe lens: *See* goniolens.

Krimsky measurement: Method of measuring a tropia in which the examiner uses prisms to move a light reflex in the patient's pupils until the reflexes are both centered.

Krukenberg's spindles: Small, round deposits of pigment on the corneal endothelium arranged in a central, vertical pattern; often associated with iritis, diabetes, and pigmentary glaucoma.

Krupin implant, shunt, or **valve:** Device implanted to control intraocular pressure by allowing aqueous fluid to flow from the anterior chamber into a filtering bleb.

L

lacri-: Root word meaning tears; *see also* dacry-.

lacrimal apparatus: Collective term for the system that produces tears and drains them from the eye; it includes the lacrimal gland and accessory lacrimal glands (which produce tear fluid), the puncta (openings inside each upper and lower eyelid through which tear fluid drains), the lacrimal ducts or canaliculi (tubules that lead to the nasolacrimal sac), the nasolacrimal sac (which holds the overflow of tears), and the nasolacrimal duct (through which tears then drain into the nasal passages).

lacrimal bone: One of the bones of the orbit.

lacrimal caruncle: Small mound of conjunctival tissue in the medial canthus.

lacrimal intubation: Surgical procedure in which a tube is implanted through the punctum, canaliculus, and nasolacrimal duct and into the nasal passage in order to restore tear drainage.

lacrimal lens: A reference to the refracting power of the tear film, generally as related to contact lens wear.

lacrimal probing: Surgical procedure in which a flexible probe is passed through the lacrimal duct in order to clear a blockage.

lacrimal sac: Another term for nasolacrimal sac.

lacrimation: Flow of tears.

lactoferrin: Protein produced by the lacrimal gland and found in tear fluid.

lactoferrin test: Test in which a filter paper is placed on the eye to absorb tear fluid, then first on a reactive plate that indicates the amount of lactoferrin present in the tears; in dry eye syndrome, lactoferrin levels are lower than normal.

lagophthalmos: Incomplete closure of eyelids, which may result in exposure keratitis.

lambda angle: *See* angle.

lamellar: Adjective describing a structure or process occurring in layers; partial-depth corneal transplants (as opposed to penetrating keratoplasty) are often described as lamellar grafts.

lamellar keratoplasty: *See* keratoplasty.

lamina cribrosa: Mesh-like area of sclera at the back of the eye through which retinal ganglion cells and blood vessels pass.

Landolt's ring: Vision test in which the optotypes are broken circles; the patient must identify the orientation of the breaks.

lase: To emit coherent light.

LASEK (laser epithelial keratomileusis): *See* keratomileusis.

laser: Acronym for *light amplification by stimulated emission of radiation*, a process invented in the early 1960s to produce coherent light; there are many types of lasers with diverse medical applications, all of which are based upon the fact that specific wavelengths of light are absorbed by specific tissues or compounds within tissues, with various consequent reactions; *see* Appendix 11; **argon l.** laser in which the light source is argon gas excited by electricity, producing laser energy in the blue-green part of the electromagnetic spectrum, which is absorbed by the red pigments of vascular tissue; action is via photocoagulation; current ophthalmic applications include treatment of diabetic retinopathy and macular degeneration, as well as trabeculoplasty and iridotomy; **carbon dioxide (CO_2) l.** laser in which the light source is carbon dioxide gas, producing laser energy at a fundamental wavelength of 10,600 nm; works via photovaporization; ophthalmic applications include removal of tumors from the orbit and cosmetic resurfacing of skin around the eyes; **diode l.** photocoagulating laser in which light is produced by electrical excitation of a solid-state semiconductor; used to treat retinal vascular disease; **dye l. (tunable dye l.)** photocoagulating laser in which a source of lased light is directed through a liquid dye that controls the wavelength of the energy that finally exits the laser; used in retinal vascular disease and glaucoma; **erbium:yttrium-aluminum-garnet (Er:YAG) l.** laser in which an Er:YAG crystal is excited by electricity and induced to emit laser light; ophthalmic applications include cosmetic procedures of the skin around the eyes and removal of cataracts; **excimer l.** photoablating laser in which the light source is an electrically excited dimer (a gas with two component elements, such as argon and fluorine); used to reshape the cornea by the process of photoablation; **helium-neon (HeNe) l.** laser producing light of a visible wavelength, used as an aiming beam for ophthalmic surgical lasers that operate at invisible wavelengths; **l. interferometer** *see* interferometer; **krypton l.** photocoagulating laser used to treat the deeper choroid; **mode-locked l.** type of Q-switched laser that employs a dye; **neodymium:yttrium-aluminum-garnet (Nd:YAG) l.** laser in which an Nd:YAG crystal is excited by electricity and induced to emit laser light of infrared wavelength; the principal ophthalmic application of the Nd:YAG laser is posterior capsulotomy, although there are applications in vitreous and glaucoma surgery; **Q-switched l.** general term for photodisrupting lasers that concentrate energy into short pulses by employing filters to prevent light from exiting the laser until a certain threshold of energy is achieved; used for "fine cutting" as in iridotomy, breaking adhesions, etc; **ruby l.** original laser using an electric arc to produce light that is made coherent by a rod composed of synthetic ruby crystal; **YAG l.** *see* Nd:YAG l.

laser in-situ keratomileusis (LASIK): *See* keratomileusis.

laser epithelial keratomileusis (LASEK): *See* keratomileusis.

laser iridotomy: Creation of a hole in the iris using a laser; performed to enhance the flow of aqueous humor, thus maintaining normal intraocular pressure in eyes suffering from or predisposed to angle-closure glaucoma.

laser reversal of presbyopia (LARP or LRP): Laser is applied to the sclera in the area of the ciliary body in order to create more tension on the zonules; *compare* surgical reversal of presbyopia (SRP).

laser trabeculoplasty: Destruction of small areas of the trabecular meshwork using a laser; performed to open the trabecular meshwork and lower intraocular pressure in eyes with glaucoma by improving aqueous outflow.

LASIK (laser in-situ keratomileusis): *See* keratomileusis.

latent: General term describing a condition that is not immediately evident, such as a phoria; *compare* manifest.

lateral: General anatomic term describing a structure or process appearing or occurring at the side, away from the midline; in ophthalmic usage, referring to the side of the eye nearest the temple; *see also* temporal; *compare* medial *and* nasal.

lateral angle: Another term for lateral canthus.

lateral canthus: Area where the upper and lower eyelids join at the side of the face nearest the temple; also called the temporal canthus and lateral angle; *compare* medial canthus.

lateral geniculate body: Area of the midbrain that receives visual impulses from the nerve fibers of the optic tract.

lateral rectus (LR) muscle: Extraocular muscle lying along the side of the eye near the temple and responsible for abducting the eye.

lattice degeneration (of the retina): Condition in which the retinal tissues thin and blood vessels harden (leading to the "lattice" appearance), with break-up of the internal limiting membrane and adhesion of the vitreous to the retina; although most eyes with lattice degeneration do not progress to retinal detachment, about one third of eyes with retinal detachments have lattice degeneration as the underlying cause.

lattice dystrophy (of the cornea): Progressive condition, usually beginning around puberty, in which lines of opacification appear through the corneal stroma and slowly increase in thickness and number.

lazy eye: Colloquial term for amblyopia; laypeople sometimes apply the term to strabismus (ie, an eye that is lazy and thus turns or drifts).

legal blindness: *See* blindness.

lens: General term for a transparent object (with two polished surfaces, at least one of them curved) that bends light rays from their original path, either to bring them together to a focus or spread them apart; *compare* prism; *see also* Bagolini l., biconcave l., biconvex l., bifocal l., bitoric l., concave l., contact l., convex l., goniolens, intraocular l., minus l., multifocal l., plus l., slab-off l., spherical l., trial l., *and* working l.; **crystalline l.** reference to the natural lens of the eye.

lens blank: Unfinished spectacle or contact lens that has not yet been ground or fabricated to its final refractive power.

lens capsule: Thin, transparent membrane surrounding the crystalline lens and to which the zonules are attached.

lens clock: Instrument used to measure the base curve of a spectacle lens; also called *Geneva lens measure.*

lens epithelium: The one-cell-thick layer of epithelial cells that covers the crystalline lens of the eye; when left in the lens capsule after cataract extraction they can proliferate to form Elschnig's pearls.

lens glide: Surgical instrument used to support and guide an intraocular lens as it is being implanted into the eye.

lens loop: Surgical instrument consisting of a handle with a small loop at the end, usually notched with small "teeth," that is used to remove the crystalline lens during extracapsular cataract extraction.

lens nucleus: *See* nucleus.

lens vault: *See* apical clearance, definition 1.

lensectomy: Surgical procedure in which the crystalline lens is removed.

lensmeter: Instrument used to measure the various components of curvature, and thus the refractive properties (ie, the "prescription") of an artificial lens.

lensometer: Another term for lensmeter.

lensometry: The act of reading a lens prescription using a lensmeter/lensometer.

lenticle: Small "button" of donor corneal tissue used in refractive keratoplasty; *see also* keratophakia.

lenticular: General term meaning of or like a lens, commonly referring to the natural crystalline lens of the eye; also used to describe "carrier" lenses for spectacle and contact lenses of high power.

lenticular astigmatism: *See* astigmatism.

lenticular cataract: Opacity of the crystalline lens; *see also* cataract.

lenticule: Alternate spelling for lenticle.

leukocoria: Literally, "white pupil," in which a dense white reflex is seen behind the pupil; associated with childhood retinoblastoma and retrolental fibroplasia.

leukoma: Dense white opacity of the cornea.

levator complex: Two-part muscle that lifts the upper eyelid, made up of the levator muscle and Müller's muscle.

levator muscle: Striated muscle portion of the levator complex that lifts the upper eyelid; more properly called the *levator palpebrae superioris*; *see also* Müller's muscle.

lid: Either of two flaps of skin that cover the eye during blinking; *see also* combining forms beginning with blephar-, palpebr-, and tars-.

lid lag: Delay in downward motion of upper eyelid when the eye looks downward; *see also* von Graefe's sign.

lid retraction: Opening of upper and/or lower lid wider than normal, resulting in excessive exposure of sclera.

lid speculum: Instrument used to hold the eyelids open.

light: Portion of the electromagnetic spectrum visible to the human eye.

light perception (LP) vision: Very low visual acuity in which the subject can perceive only the presence or absence of light and is unable to see objects; *see also* count-finger vision, hand-motion vision, light projection vision, no light perception vision, *and* visual acuity.

light projection (LP w/proj) vision: Low visual acuity in which the subject cannot see objects but can perceive not only the presence of light (ie, light perception), but also the direction from which it is shining.

limbal: General medical term meaning near the line along which two structures meet; in ophthalmic usage, usually referring to the circular border between the cornea and sclera.

limbal conjunctiva: *See* conjunctiva.

limbus: General anatomic term for the line along which two structures meet; most commonly in ophthalmic usage, the circular border between the cornea and sclera.

limiting membranes (of retina): *See* retina.

line(s) of visual acuity: Reference to Snellen's visual acuity measurement in which the notation for distance visual acuity ranges from very low (20/400) to "normal" (20/20) and corresponds to lines of letters of diminishing size on the test chart; for example, a change from 20/20 to 20/30 visual acuity would be described as a "one-line loss," a change from 20/30 to 20/60 would be a "three-line loss," etc.

lipid layer: Outer layer of the tear film consisting of oily secretions produced in the meibomian glands; *see also* tear film.

loop: *See* lens loop.

loupe: Low-power magnifying device for viewing objects at very close range; usually referring to two loupes attached to a spectacle frame, employed by professionals performing close work on small objects (eg, jeweler's loupes) or by low-vision patients; before the operating microscope came into wide use, the patient's eye would be viewed during surgery through loupes worn by the surgeon.

low-pressure or **low-tension glaucoma:** *See* glaucoma.

low vision (LV): Visual impairment that cannot be remedied with corrective lenses or surgical intervention, usually describing a condition in which bilateral retinal pathology (eg, macular degeneration) renders an individual unable to perform normal daily functions; low vision is not synonymous with legal blindness; low vision has no objective definition because people have such widely varying needs for near versus distance vision or the ability to discern colors or fine detail.

low vision aids: General term for devices designed to help low-vision patients perform their daily tasks; *see* bioptics, loupe, magnifier, telescope, *and* typoscope.

lubricant: Substance designed to moisturize.

lumen: 1. General term for the hollow area inside a duct or tube (eg, the lumen of the lacrimal duct); 2. in optics, the standard unit of the amount of light flowing through a solid angle (ie, a space shaped like a cone); one lumen (1 lm) is defined as the flux of light through one steradian emitted by a light source with one candela intensity.

M

macrophthalmia, -os: Condition in which the eyeball is abnormally large; *compare* microphthalmia.

macropia, -sia: Visual defect in which objects appear larger than they really are; *compare* micropia.

macula: General anatomic term derived from the Latin for spot or stain; most commonly in ophthalmic usage, the small yellowish area of the retina where cone cells are most densely packed (more properly called the *macula luteae*); it is usually just below and temporal to the optic disk; the center of the macula is slightly depressed and known as the *fovea*, which in turn has a pit at its center called the *foveola*; **corneal m.** area of cloudiness or white opacity on the cornea; **false m.** area of the retina that has an anomalous retinal correspondence with the macula of the fixating eye; *see* anomalous retinal correspondence.

macular degeneration (MD): General term for conditions in which the macular tissue breaks down, resulting in a loss of central vision; the visual loss is generally irreversible, although vitamin therapy, laser treatment, and surgical therapies are employed to slow its progression; **age-related m.d. (ARMD)** macular degeneration resulting from age-related changes in the small blood vessels, nerve cells, pigment epithelium, and other tissues in the macula; **dry m.d.** relatively mild form of macular degeneration that is not accompanied by the formation of retinal exudates; *compare* wet m.d.; **senile m.d. (SMD)** another term for age-related m.d.; **wet m.d.** more severe form of macular degeneration that is accompanied by the formation of retinal exudates as a result of new, abnormal blood vessel growth (choroidal neovascularization).

macular hole: A small, well-defined opening in the macula through the entire thickness of the retina, possibly as a result of the vitreous body pulling on its attachments in the area of the macula.

macular pucker: *See* epiretinal membrane.

macular sparing: Condition in which the central vision remains functional although the rest of the field exhibits extensive damage; seen in lesions affecting the optic radiations or the occipital lobe of the brain.

macular splitting: Condition in which the left or right side of the visual field, including the central field, is divided (ie, half of the field, specifically including the central field, remains).

maculopathy: General term for disorders of the macula.

Maddox rod: A red lens composed of cylinders; a point source of light viewed through the Maddox rod appears as a red streak of light; used in measuring muscle deviations, especially phorias.

magnetic resonance imaging (MRI): Use of radio waves (created by a strong magnetic field) to create an image of the body's interior; best used to view soft tissues; in ophthalmology, used to evaluate conditions involving swelling, tumors, and nerves; *compare* computerized tomography.

magnifier: In ophthalmic usage, a device used by low-vision patients to enlarge objects for better viewing, usually to facilitate reading and writing; **hand-held m.** magnifier consisting of a high-power plus lens that is held by the user; **projection m.** magnifier that projects an enlarged image of the object to be viewed onto a screen; **stand m.** magnifier consisting of a high-power plus lens that is mounted on a stand, leaving the user's hands free.

magnify: To visually enlarge, generally by the use of plus spherical lenses; *compare* minify.

malar bone: Another name for the zygomatic bone, one of the bones of the orbit.

malignant glaucoma: *See* glaucoma.

malignant myopia: *See* degenerative myopia *under* myopia.

malingering: Situation in which the patient purposely gives false information (usually to make the vision, etc, appear worse than it is) during subjective testing in order to gain something (financial reimbursement, a pair of glasses, sympathy, etc); includes memorizing the eye chart to make vision seem better than it is (to get drivers license, a job, etc).

manifest: General term describing a condition that is evident, such as a tropia; *compare* latent.

manifest refraction (MR): 1. Determining the refractive error at distance vision so that the eye does not accommodate but without using drugs that actually prevent accommodation; 2. the refractive error measured in this manner.

manual vitrectomy: *See* vitrectomy.

Marcus Gunn pupil: Impairment of the normal response of the affected pupil to bright light when stimulated by the light; verified by the swinging flashlight test, in which the examiner shines a light first into one eye, then into the other, then again into the first, comparing the response of the two pupils; Marcus Gunn pupil usually appears as a constriction of both pupils when the unaffected eye is illuminated, followed by an apparent dilation of both pupils when the affected eye is illuminated; the defect is sometimes manifest by the affected pupil constricting *less* to a direct light stimulus than does the unaffected pupil when presented with the same stimulus; also called *afferent pupillary defect*; **reverse M.G.p.** situation in which the pupil of the affected eye is fixed; during the swinging flashlight test, the unaffected pupil will dilate when the light is shown into the affected pupil; when the light is swung to the unaffected pupil, that pupil will constrict very rapidly.

mast cell: Cell (present in various tissues including those of the eye) that plays a role in the release of histamine and other substances involved in allergy; **m.c. stabilizer** in ophthalmic usage, a topical drug that acts to prevent mast cells from releasing histamines, and thus prevent or diminish the severity of ocular allergies.

maxillary bone: One of the bones of the orbit.

medial: General anatomic term describing a structure or process appearing or occurring in the middle; in ophthalmic usage, referring to the area of the eye nearest the nose; *see also* nasal; *compare* lateral *and* temporal.

medial angle: Another term for medial canthus.

medial canthus: Area where the upper and lower eyelids join at the side of the face nearest the nose; also called the *medial angle; compare* lateral canthus.

medial rectus (MR) muscle: Extraocular muscle lying along the side of the eye near the nose and responsible for adducting the eye.

medium, -ia: In optical usage, transparent object(s) or substance(s) through which light travels; the fact that light travels at different speeds in different substances accounts for the different degrees to which light is bent (refracted) by various media; *see also* refractive index; **ocular m.** or **refracting m.** tissues in the eye through which light is transmitted: the cornea, aqueous humor, lens, and vitreous humor; sometimes includes the tear film.

megalophthalmia, -os: Another term for macrophthalmia.

megalopia, -sia: Another term for macropia.

meibomian cyst: Inflammation of the eyelid that results in the collection of fluid within the meibomian glands; may develop into a chalazion; *see also* hordeolum.

meibomian glands: Glands located within the eyelids that produce oil; their secretions form the outer layer of the tear film; also called the *tarsal glands*.

meibomianitis or **meibomitis:** Inflammation of the meibomian glands.

melting: *See* corneal melting.

membrane: General medical term for a thin tissue layer that acts as a "skin" or covering, lining, or connection between tissues, either as part of normal anatomy or a disease process; *see also* Bruch's m., choroidal neovascular m., cyclitic m., Descemet's m., epiretinal m., hyaloid m., *and* preretinal m.; **anterior basal m.** *see* Bowman's capsule; **anterior hyaloid m.** *see* hyaloid membrane; **basement m.** general medical term for the thin membrane that lies underneath the epithelium of certain tissues; in ophthalmic practice often referring to the basement membrane of the choroid and corneal epithelium.

membranectomy: Surgical removal of a membrane; in ophthalmic usage, usually referring to removal of retinal membranes.

meniscus lens: Another term for convexoconcave lens.

meridian: Geometric term for a line passing through the poles (two points diametrically opposite) of a sphere; in ophthalmic usage: 1. standard reference lines used to describe positions on the eyeball; 2. used to describe the positions of the greatest and least curvature, generally on the cornea or a contact lens.

meshwork: *See* trabecular meshwork.

mesopia: Vision under conditions of partial lighting, such as dimly lit rooms or outdoors at sunset and sunrise; *compare* photopia *and* scotopia.

methylcellulose: Organic compound that is a component of some artificial tears and viscoelastic substances.

microphthalmia, -os: Abnormally small eye; *compare* macrophthalmia.

micropia, -sia: Visual defect in which objects appear smaller than they really are; *compare* macropia.

microsaccades: Extremely fine involuntary movements of the eye that occur while the eye is fixated on an object; *see also* saccades.

microscope: Optical instrument that uses lenses to magnify objects; **biomicroscope** another term for slit lamp m.; **operating m.** microscope used by the ophthalmic surgeon to obtain an enlarged view of the eye; it is typically outfitted with a bright light and often has multiple eyepieces for use by other personnel or attachment of a camera; **slit lamp m.** *see* slit lamp.

microstrabismus: *See* strabismus.

minify: To decrease the apparent size of an object, usually with minus spherical lenses; *compare* magnify.

minus: 1. Property of an optical system such that it causes rays of light to diverge (eg, a biconcave lens); 2. in spoken ophthalmic usage, synonym for myopia (eg, a "minus 2 diopter patient").

minus lens: Lens that causes incoming rays of light to diverge (*see* concave lens *and* cylinder, definition 2); in common ophthalmic usage, the power of the minus sphere lens used to correct nearsightedness is often used to describe the degree of myopia (thus, a "high minus" or "minus six" patient).

miosis: Constriction of one or both pupils in response to stimulation by bright light, to accommodation, or to certain drugs or disease processes; *compare* mydriasis.

miotic: 1. State in which one or both pupils are constricted (generally meaning 2 mm or smaller); 2. any process or agent that constricts the pupils (as in a miotic drug).

mire: General term for a reference line of standard shape on a measuring device (eg, lensometer, keratometer, etc).

mixed astigmatism: *See* astigmatism.

Miyake photography or **view:** Method for viewing the anterior segment of a cadaver eye from the rear by dissecting the front part of the eye and fixing it to a clear plate, behind which the camera is located.

model eye: *See* schematic eye.

modulation transfer function: Laboratory method for determining the light-transmitting characteristics of an optical system by analyzing light of known wave form after it passes through the system.

monochromatism: Condition in which only one of the three visual pigments is present, usually cyanolabe; *compare* achromatism, dichromatism, *and* trichromatism.

monocular: Literally, "one eyed;" used alone to describe a patient with one eye or combined with another term to describe an ocular condition involving only one eye, as in monocular vision (ie, seeing with only one eye), monocular diplopia (ie, double image in one eye), etc; *compare* binocular.

monovision: Situation in which one eye sees at near and the other at distance, usually artificially created for the presbyope using either contact lenses or intraocular lens implants.

morgagnian cataract: *See* cataract.

motor fusion: *See* fusion.

mucin: Protein that is the primary component of mucus; in the eye, goblet cells in the conjunctiva produce the mucin that is found in tear fluid.

Mueller's cells: Retinal cells located in the inner nuclear layer with fibers extending to the internal and external limiting membranes; Mueller's cells serve as part of the structural meshwork of the retina and supply nutrients and other metabolic materials to retinal nerve cells.

Müller's muscle: Smooth muscle portion of the levator complex that opens the upper lid; also called the *superior tarsal muscle; see also* levator muscle.

multifocal lens: Artificial lens that is designed to provide more than one, and usually more than two, focal points; several multifocal systems have been developed for spectacle, intraocular, and contact lenses; *see also* aspheric, bifocal lens, *and* diffractive multifocal lens.

multiple vision: General term for visual defect in which a single object is perceived as several images; *see also* diplopia.

mutton-fat precipitates: *See* keratic precipitates.

myasthenia gravis (MG): Chronic systemic disease characterized by muscle weakness; in the eye, ptosis and diplopia are typical.

mydriasis: Widening of one or both pupils, usually as a response to reduced light but also to certain drugs or disease processes; *see also* dilation; *compare* miosis.

mydriatic: Condition or agent that dilates the pupils, as in a mydriatic drug.

myope: Individual with myopia.

myotonic pupil: Another term for *tonic pupil*.

myopia: Another term for nearsightedness; refractive error in which the eye focuses rays of light so that the focal point is in front of the retina, with the result that distant objects are not clearly seen; **axial m.** nearsightedness attributable to the length of the eye (ie, the eye is too long for images to be focused on the retina); **degenerative m.** nearsightedness attributable to severe, ongoing structural changes in the eye, eventually resulting in permanent damage to the retina; **high m.** nonspecific term for extreme myopia beyond what is found in most of the population, usually referring to myopia of -6 diopters or greater; **lenticular m.** nearsightedness attributable to excessive (plus) power of the crystalline lens; **low m.** nonspecific term for small amount of myopia, usually referring to myopia of -2 diopters or less; **malignant m.** *see* degenerative m.; **moderate m.** nonspecific term referring to an amount of myopia that causes significant but not extreme visual impairment, usually referring to myopia between -2 and -6 diopters; **night m.** difficulty seeing at a distance in dim light, occurring because the dilated pupil reduces the depth of field; **progressive m.** nearsightedness that continues to worsen; **refractive m.** nearsightedness that is attributable to the refractive power of the eye (ie, the refractive power of the cornea and lens is too great and brings incoming rays of light to focus in front of the retina); *compare* axial m.; **school m.** nearsightedness that seems to arise from prolonged use of near vision for reading during the school year.

myopic keratomileusis: *See* keratomileusis.

N

nanophthalmia, -os: Another term for microphthalmia.

narrow-angle glaucoma (NAG): *See* closed-angle glaucoma *under* glaucoma.

nasal: General anatomic directional term meaning toward the nose; *see also* medial; *compare* lateral *and* temporal.

nasal bone: Either of two bones lying between the orbits and forming the bridge of the nose.

nasal canthus: Another term for medial canthus.

nasal step: Visual field defect in which a two-part defect "steps" from nasal to temporal with a normal field in between; corresponds to damage of nerve fibers near the central portion of the retina's nasal side; most often associated with glaucoma.

nasolacrimal duct (NLD): Canal through which tear fluid drains from the nasolacrimal sac into the nasal passages; *see also* lacrimal apparatus.

nasolacrimal sac: Internal sac adjacent to the eye that holds tears that have drained off the eye.

near point of accommodation (NPA): Distance from the eye to the nearest point clearly visible when accommodation is at its maximum.

near point of convergence (NPC): Nearest point where the eyes can maintain binocular vision by pulling together; the greatest degree of convergence that the eyes can attain.

near vision: The distance at which visual tasks such as reading are performed, generally defined to be about 14 to 16 inches; *compare* distance vision; *see also* vision.

nearsightedness: Another term for myopia.

neovascular glaucoma: *See* glaucoma.

neovascularization: Abnormal growth of blood vessels caused by some disorder or disease state, most often seen in diabetic retinopathy; these new vessels are generally weak and prone to leakage and bleeding; **corneal n.** abnormal blood vessel growth into the cornea, usually associated with contact lens wear; **retinal n.** abnormal blood vessel growth into the retina, usually associated with diabetes and hypertension.

nerve fiber layer (NFL): Retinal nerve fibers (actually, axons of the ganglion cell layer) that come together at the optic nerve head; their unique pattern of distribution plays a key role in the appearance of visual field defects, most notably in glaucoma; *see also* retina.

neuro-ophthalmology: Medical subspecialty concerned with the nervous system's involvement with the eye, both sensory and motor; includes ocular movements, pupillary responses, and the structures of the brain involved in vision.

neurotransmitter: Biochemical that crosses the gap between nerve cells, attaches to specific receptor sites, and thus carries messages from the brain; *see* acetylcholine, epinephrine, *and* norepinephrine.

neutralization: 1. In optics, act of determining the power of an unknown lens; *see also* lensometry; 2. in retinoscopy, act of determining the refractive state of the eye by adjusting lenses before the eye until the pupil is uniformly illuminated by the retinoscope; 3. act of correcting a refractive error with lenses or strabismus with prisms.

nevus: A nonmalignant lesion on the skin or other tissue; may or may not be pigmented and/or raised and/or smooth; in the eye, it is more frequently found on the lids, conjunctiva, iris, and choroid, but can appear on other tissues/structures as well; plural: nevi.

nictitation: Blinking, especially in animals that have a thin, translucent membrane (ie, nictitating membrane) instead of fleshy eyelids.

night blindness: Another term for nyctalopia.

night vision: *See* scotopia.

no light perception (NLP) vision: Total blindness; *see also* count-finger vision, hand-motion vision, light perception vision, *and* visual acuity.

nocturnal amblyopia: *See* nyctalopia.

nodal point: Another term for optical center.

nomogram: A mathematical formula or graph used to calculate necessary action for a specific outcome; ocular procedures using nomograms include contact lens fitting, intraocular lens selection, refractive surgery methods (ie, how many incisions, how deep, and where to place them; size of pupillary zone; how much tissue to remove; etc); such a formula or graph that allows each practitioner or surgeon to enter numbers specific to his or her own methods, experience, and other data that will enable the best results.

nonaccommodative esotropia: *See* esotropia.

nonconcomitant: Another term for incomitant.

noncontact tonometer: Instrument that measures intraocular pressure without actually touching the eye; *see also* pneumotonometer *under* tonometer.

nondominant eye: The eye that is subjectively less preferred for use by an individual, much the way one hand is less preferred than the other; *compare* dominant eye.

nonsteroidal anti-inflammatory drug (NSAID): A drug used to reduce inflammation that does not contain steroids, thus avoiding the undesirable side effects of steroids; *see* corticosteroid.

noradrenaline: Another term for norepinephrine.

norepinephrine: One of two biochemicals that conducts messages for the sympathetic nervous system (the other is epinephrine); *compare* acetylcholine.

normal retinal correspondence (NRC): *See* retinal correspondence.

Nu value: Another term for *Abbe value*.

nuclear adhesions: Small areas where the nucleus and cortex of the crystalline lens normally are attached.

nuclear cataract: *See* cataract.

nuclear layer (of the retina): One of two layers of retinal nerve tissue; the outer nuclear (or bacillary) layer consists of the rod and cone cells, and the inner layer consists of the amacrine and bipolar cells, as well as the capillaries that carry blood through the retina; *see also* retina.

nucleus: General term for a central structure; in ophthalmic usage, most commonly referring to the nucleus of the crystalline lens.

nyctalope: Individual with nyctalopia.

nyctalopia: Visual defect in which vision is greatly reduced in low light conditions, most often as a result of retinal pigment insufficiency; commonly called *night blindness*.

nystagmus: Rapid, rhythmic, involuntary eye movements; nystagmus is classified according to the direction of motion (horizontal is the most common) and the stimuli that cause it to occur; *see* Appendix 5; **amaurotic n.** nystagmus of a blind eye; **caloric n.** nonpathological nystagmus that results when warm or cold fluid is introduced into the ear; **conjugate n.** nystagmus in which the eyes move in the same direction and with the same rhythm; **disconjugate n.** nystagmus in which the eyes exhibit different directions or rhythms; **dissociated n.** nystagmus in which the amplitude of the movements are not the same in both eyes; **endpoint n.** nonpathological nystagmus that sometimes occurs when the eyes are turned as far in one direction as possible; **fixation n.** nystagmus that occurs as the eyes attempt to maintain prolonged fixation; **jerk n.** another term for rhythmic n.; **labyrinthine n.** another term for caloric n.; **latent n.** nystagmus that either appears or increases when one eye is covered; **optokinetic n. (OKN)** nonpathological, rapid movements of the eyes as they move to fixate on rhythmic, repeating stimuli; also called *railroad n.*; **pendular n.** nystagmus in which the eye's movement in one direction is equal to the movement in the other; **physiologic n.** nonpathological nystagmus that can be evoked in the normal person; **rhythmic n.** pattern of eye movement that is slower in one direction followed by a more rapid movement back to the original position; **rotatory n.** nystagmus in which the eyes revolve around the visual axis; **vestibular n.** another term for caloric n.

O

objective: Method of testing that does not require input from the patient (examples: retinoscopy, Krimsky measurement, slit lamp exam); *compare* subjective.

objective lens: In optical systems, especially telescopes and microscopes, the lens nearest to the object being viewed; *compare* ocular.

obligatory suppression: Constant mental "blocking out" of the image from one eye in order to prevent double vision, whether the eye is deviated or not; *compare* facultative suppression.

oblique astigmatism: *See* astigmatism.

oblique muscles: *See* inferior oblique muscle *and* superior oblique muscle.

O'Brien block: Injection of anesthetic agents to achieve akinesia (prevention of movement) of the eyelids.

occluder: Opaque instrument, lens, or patch used to cover one eye during ophthalmic testing.

occlusion: General term for blockage or closing; 1. in most common ophthalmic usage, covering an eye, typically during a vision examination; **o. therapy** treatment for amblyopia that involves patching the strong eye in order to force the weak eye to work; 2. in surgery the blockage of the aspiration port of an irrigation and aspiration probe.

occupational bifocal or **segment:** Multifocal lens with a near segment at the top instead of the bottom, designed to provide close vision overhead.

Occupational Safety and Health Administration (OSHA): Governmental agency that establishes and enforces standards regarding the safety and health of employees; in part, these standards are designed to reduce/eliminate risks associated with exposure to harmful pathogens (such as hepatitis and human immunodeficiency virus [HIV]).

ocul-: Combining form meaning eye.

ocular: 1. General anatomic adjective meaning of or related to the eye (eg, ocular testing, ocular surgery, etc); 2. eyepiece of a microscope or other optical instrument; *compare* objective lens.

ocular adnexa: *See* adnexa.

ocular angle: Another term for canthus.

ocular hypertension (OHT): High intraocular pressure (IOP); IOP of 20 to 22 millimeters of mercury (mmHg) is generally considered the border between "normal" IOP and ocular hypertension in otherwise healthy eyes; ocular hypertension is not the same as glaucoma because glaucoma only exists if there is some indication of damage; *see also* glaucoma suspect *and* intraocular pressure.

ocular media: Tissues in the eye through which light is transmitted: the cornea, aqueous humor, lens, and vitreous humor.

ocular motility: General term for the processes by which the eyes move in a controlled, coordinated fashion, or the study of the function and disorders of alignment and movement of the eyes.

ocular pemphigoid: *See* pemphigoid.

ocular prosthesis: Artificial device resembling the eye that is placed in the socket after surgical removal of the eye (correct clinical term for "glass eye"); *compare* orbital implant.

ocularist: Individual trained to make and fit ocular prostheses.

oculi uterque: Latin phrase meaning either or both eyes, abbreviation for which (OU) is commonly used in ophthalmic speech and literature.

oculogyration: Circular motion or rotation of the eyes.

oculomotor: General term referring to eye movement and the muscle and nerve systems that initiate and control it.

oculomotor nerve: The third cranial nerve, which innervates the extraocular muscles except the superior oblique and lateral rectus.

oculopathy: General term for unhealthy condition of the eye.

oculoplastics: Surgical specialty concerned with reconstructive and cosmetic surgery of the orbit, eyelids, and ocular adnexa.

oculopupillary reflex: Dilation of the pupils when the surface of the eyeball or eyelids is touched or irritated.

oculus dexter: Latin phrase meaning right eye, abbreviation for which (OD) is commonly used in ophthalmic speech and literature.

oculus sinister: Latin phrase meaning left eye, abbreviation for which (OS) is commonly used in ophthalmic speech and literature.

onchocerciasis: Condition in which a small parasitic worm infests the skin, connective tissues, and eyes of its host; a significant cause of blindness in areas of the world where clean water is not always available; also known as *river blindness*; *see also* filariasis.

-op-, -opt-: Combining form meaning see or sight.

open-angle glaucoma: *See* glaucoma.

open-sky: General term for surgical procedures (usually vitrectomy) in which the whole cornea is removed to give the surgeon access to the internal structures of the eye; this very traumatic approach has been abandoned in most contemporary ophthalmic surgery.

operating microscope: *See* microscope.

operculated retinal hole or **tear:** Retinal hole in which a piece of retinal tissue is separated around its entire circumference and pulled away from the surrounding retina by its attachment to the vitreous body.

ophthalm-: Combining form meaning eye.

ophthalmalgia: Eye pain.

ophthalmia: General term for inflammation of the eye; *see also* sympathetic ophthalmia; **o. neonatorum** *see* conjunctivitis.

ophthalmic: Related to or involving the eye (eg, ophthalmic surgery or ophthalmic disease).

ophthalmic artery: Main vessel bringing blood into the eye and orbit, entering the optic foramen, and dividing into vessels that enter the retina, lacrimal apparatus, extraocular muscles, etc.

ophthalmic medical personnel (OMP): Person trained to assist an ophthalmologist; three certification levels and several subspecialties are available; *see* Appendix 19.

ophthalmitis: General term for inflammation of the eye.

ophthalmodynamometry (ODM): Technique for measuring blood pressure in the central retinal artery by applying pressure to the sclera until the artery can be seen to stop pulsating (via ophthalmoscopy).

ophthalmologist: Medical doctor (MD degree from an accredited medical school) specializing in care of the eye, including correction of refractive errors, diagnosis, and both pharmacological and surgical treatments.

ophthalmometer: General term for any instrument that measures the state of the eye; most commonly in ophthalmic usage referring to a keratometer.

ophthalmopathy: General term for disease of the eye.

ophthalmoplegia: Paralysis of the eye.

ophthalmoscope: Instrument for viewing the inside of the eye; **binocular o.** ophthalmoscope that allows the examiner to use both eyes when viewing a subject's eye, thereby obtaining a three-dimensional image; *see also* direct ophthalmoscopy *and* indirect ophthalmoscopy.

opsoclonia: Involuntary, arrhythmic, rapid movements of the eyes, usually resulting from injury or insult to the brain.

optic: 1. Related to or involving vision or the eye (eg, optic nerve); 2. an element of an optical system (eg, a lens or prism); 3. the central focusing portion of an intraocular lens; *compare* haptic.

optic atrophy: Degeneration of nerve fibers in the optic disk, described in its two major manifestations as primary and secondary optic atrophy.

optic chiasm: Point at which the two optic nerves meet; the nasal nerve fibers from each eye cross here, while the temporal fibers continue on the same side; the impulses from the right and left sides of the retina of each eye are directed to the geniculate body and the occipital lobe in such a way that the right brain receives and fuses the right sides of the two retinal images and the left brain receives the left sides; also called *optic nerve decussation*.

optic cup: *See* cup.

optic disk: Roughly circular area at the back of the eye where nerve fibers converge to form the optic nerve, creating a "blind spot" where images are not perceived; also called *optic nerve head*; *see also* physiologic scotoma *under* scotoma.

optic foramen: Opening in the orbit (eye socket of the skull) through which the optic nerve passes.

optic nerve (ON): The bundle of retinal nerve fibers that exits each eye; the optic nerves meet at the optic chiasm.

optic nerve head: Another term for *optic disk*.

optical: Related to or involving a system through which light is transmitted.

optical axis: *See* axis.

optical center (OC): Point of a lens through which a ray of light may pass without being bent (ie, refracted); also called the *nodal point of a lens*; the OC of a lens is generally aligned with the patient's optical axis (line of sight).

optical zone (OZ): Area of a lens or tissue through which the eye sees; used in describing corrective spectacle, contact, or intraocular lenses to designate the optically functioning part of the lens from structural or other parts; in corneal refractive surgery, the portion of the cornea that is intended to provide the refractive correction.

optician: Individual trained to make vision correcting lenses and to dispense and adjust eyewear.

optics: Study of the nature and behavior of light; for important optical principles, *see* electromagnetic spectrum, focus, lens, light, prism, reflection, *and* refraction.

optometrist: Doctor of optometry (OD degree from an accredited school of optometry) trained in the diagnosis and treatment of refractive errors and medical conditions of the eye, with some training in general medical principles; most are authorized (depending on their state's optometric practice laws) to use some prescription pharmaceuticals in diagnosis and treatment of ocular conditions; with very few highly controversial exceptions, no state authorizes optometrists to perform any type of surgery, including laser surgery.

optotype: General term for standardized image used in visual acuity tests (derived from Snellen's term for the letters on his original chart).

ora serrata: Irregular anterior border of the retina where it attaches to the choroid, located adjacent to the pars plana of the ciliary body and approximately 8 mm posterior to the corneoscleral limbus.

orb: In ophthalmic usage, the eyeball.

orbicularis oculi muscle: Muscle that controls blinking and closure of the eyelids; it encircles the eye with fibers in the upper and lower lids.

orbit: Either of two spherical hollows in the skull that protect and provide attachments for the eyes, extraocular muscles, and surrounding tissues; commonly known as the *eye socket*, the orbit consists of the ethmoid, frontal, lacrimal, maxillary, palatine, sphenoid, and zygomatic bones.

orbital crest: Area of the skull just above the orbit at the level of the eyebrow.

orbital decompression: Surgical procedure to increase the volume of the orbit by removing bone from its wall and thus relieve pressure on the eye, usually in treatment of an ocular tumor.

orbital fissure: One of two openings (superior and inferior) in each orbit through which blood vessels and nerves pass.

orbital implant: Biologically inert device implanted in the orbit and under the conjunctiva after enucleation in order to maintain the volume of the orbit; also called *enucleation implant*; *compare* ocular prosthesis.

orthokeratology (ortho-K): Treatment of refractive error by prescribing rigid contact lenses designed to gradually reshape the cornea.

orthophoria: Normal state in which the eyes remain properly oriented even if one or the other is occluded; *see also* phoria; *compare* heterophoria.

orthoptics: System for nonsurgical correction of strabismus and other defects of ocular motility; *see also* vision training.

oscillating vision: Another term for oscillopsia.

oscillopsia: State in which objects appear to move back and forth.

OSHA: *See* Occupational Safety and Health Administration.

osmotic: General chemical term for a process or agent that influences the flow of liquids across a membrane; in ophthalmic usage, osmotics are used topically or systemically to draw water out of the eye, thus reducing intraocular pressure.

outer granular or **outer granular layer (of retina):** Cell layer within the retina where the synapses of the outer and inner nuclear layers meet; *see also* retina.

outer limiting membrane (of retina): *See* external limiting membrane (of retina).

outer nuclear layer (of retina): Cell layer within the retina composed primarily of bipolar cells and containing the rod and cone cell bodies, located between the inner and outer molecular layers; *see also* retina.

outflow: In ophthalmic usage, the drainage either of tears through the puncta into the nasolacrimal system or of aqueous humor from the anterior chamber into Schlemm's canal.

overcorrection: Excessive correction of refractive error, making a nearsighted eye farsighted or a farsighted eye nearsighted, usually referring to a refractive surgical procedure or intraocular lens implantation that missed its intended target; *compare* undercorrection.

over-refraction: Technique of determining the amount of corrective power needed in addition to the corrective lenses currently in place; determined by using an autorefractor or phoropter to perform refractometry while the patient wears eyeglasses or contact lenses.

P

pachymetry: Measurement of the thickness of the cornea; the instrument used to make the measurement is a *pachymeter*.

palatine bone: One of the bones of the orbit.

pallor: General term for abnormal whiteness (paleness) of tissue; in ophthalmic usage, change in color of the optic disk from yellow to white, indicative of retinal damage (as in glaucoma).

palpebra: Proper medical term for the eyelid; plural: palpebrae; **inferior p.** lower eyelid; **superior p.** upper eyelid.

palpebral conjunctiva: Mucosal tissue lining the inner surface of the eyelids; *see also* conjunctiva; *compare* bulbar conjunctiva.

palpebral fissure: The gap between the upper and lower eyelids.

pannus: In ophthalmic usage, condition in which blood vessels grow into the cornea, which then becomes fibrous and loses its transparency; may be classified according to type as allergic, glaucomatous, etc.

panophthalmitis: Widespread inflammation of the tissues of the eye.

panretinal photocoagulation: Laser surgical procedure in which laser energy is applied across wide areas of the retina in an attempt to stop the progression of retinopathy.

pantoscopic tilt: Fit of spectacles so that the bottom of the frame front is angled closer to the cheeks; ideal is between 4 and 18 degrees; *compare* retroscopic tilt.

Panum's fusion area or **fusional space:** Area in front of and behind the horopter where fusion occurs, making stereopsis possible; *see also* horopter.

papilla: Small nodular elevation on a tissue; plural: papillae; **lacrimal p.** slightly elevated area on the edge of the eyelid, near the nose, where the punctum is located; **optic p.** *see* optic disk.

papillae: In ophthalmic usage, small elevated areas of palpebral conjunctiva with central blood vessels, present in conjunctival infection or allergy.

papillary conjunctivitis: *See* conjunctivitis: giant papillary.

papilledema: Noninflammatory swelling of the optic disk with engorgement of blood vessels as a result of increased intracranial pressure, malignant hypertension, or central retinal vein occlusion; also called *choked disk.*

papillomacular bundle: Dense, oval bundle of retinal nerve ganglion cell fibers extending from the macula into the central optic nerve.

paracentesis: General term for a surgical technique that involves an incision into a fluid-filled cavity; in ophthalmic usage, an incision into the anterior chamber of the eye.

paracentral scotoma: *See* scotoma.

paradoxical: General term describing a sign or symptom, such as visual field loss or diplopia, that has a peculiar feature or is of uncertain cause.

parakinesia: In ophthalmic usage, general term for abnormal motor function of the muscles of the eye.

parallax: Optical phenomenon in which an object shifts in the field of view when the observer changes position; nearer objects appear to shift opposite to the direction of the observer's head while distant objects seem to move in the same direction; **binocular p.** a shift in the relative position of objects when the observer views first with one eye alone and then with the other eye alone.

paraoptometric: Personnel trained to assist an optometrist; three certification levels are available; *see* Appendix 19.

parasympathetic nervous system: Division of the autonomic nervous system that encourages digestion and maintains energy reserves; in the eye, this system causes pupil miosis and accommodation; *see also* acetylcholine; *compare* sympathetic nervous system.

parasympatholytic: Substance that blocks the parasympathetic system, thus causing a sympathetic response; also called *cholinergic-blocking*; cyclopentolate (a cycloplegic) is an example; *compare* sympatholytic.

parasympathomimetic: Substance that causes a parasympathetic-like response; also called *cholinergic*; pilocarpine (a miotic) is an example; *compare* sympathomimetic.

parophthalmia: Inflammation of the tissues surrounding the eye.

pars: General anatomic term meaning part.

pars plana: Commonly used term for the outermost ring of the ciliary body (more properly called the *pars plana corporis ciliaris*); vitrectomy is sometimes carried out through an incision at the level of the pars plana.

pars plicata: The innermost ring of the ciliary body consisting of the ciliary processes.

passive forced duction test: Another term for forced duction test.

pemphigoid: In ophthalmic usage, a condition in which the conjunctiva blisters, leading to dryness of the eye and adhesion to the eyelids.

penetrating keratoplasty: Surgical procedure in which the entire cornea is removed and replaced with donated tissue, popularly known as *corneal transplantation*; *see also* keratoplasty.

perfluorocarbon: Class of heavy gases, such as perfluoropropane (C_3F_8), used in retinal detachment repair; *see also* gas-fluid exchange.

perforation: Piercing of a tissue or structure, usually as a result of trauma or a complication of surgery.

peribulbar: Term describing the area around the eye.

peribulbar anesthesia: Anesthesia administered in several injections around the periphery of the eyeball; *compare* retrobulbar anesthesia.

perimeter: In ophthalmic usage, an instrument used to perform perimetry (visual field testing).

perimetry: Technique of visual field testing that determines the boundaries of the field of view by presenting test targets (most often points of light) to the test subject, who fixates upon the middle of a blank screen and reports when the target becomes visible in the periphery; **automated p.** perimetry in which a computer assists in selecting and recording the position of targets and provides a printout of the test results (also called *computerized perimetry*); **Goldmann p.** perimetry in which a machine controlled by an examiner is used to map out the visual field (vs. automated, where a computer performs this function); results are recorded manually; **kinetic p.** perimetry in which the target moves from the periphery of the visual field toward the central fixation point until the subject reports that it is visible; **manual p.** perimetry that is controlled by an examiner (eg, Goldmann p., tangent screen); **static p.** perimetry in which the target is a stationary point of light that gradually increases in brightness until the subject reports that it is visible.

periodic strabismus: *See* strabismus.

periorbital: Near the eye or the bony eye socket.

peripheral cataract: *See* cataract.

peripheral iridectomy: *See* iridectomy.

peripheral vision: Perception of objects in the outer areas of the field of view.

peritomy: In ophthalmic usage, an incision into the conjunctiva at the limbus; also called *peritectomy*.

persistence of vision: *See* afterimage.

phaco- or **phako-:** Combining form meaning lens, usually referring to the natural crystalline lens of the eye but also applicable to artificial lenses; note that in British usage, phako- is the only acceptable combining form.

phaco: *See* phacoemulsification.

phacoablation: A still-experimental surgical technique of cataract removal by which lens tissue is vaporized by the action of a laser.

phacoanaphylaxis: Condition in which leakage of proteins from the crystalline lens leads to inflammation within the eye.

phacodonesis: Movement of the crystalline lens, usually as a result of broken zonules.

phacoemulsification (phaco): Surgical technique for cataract extraction using a probe that vibrates at ultrasonic frequency (approximately 40,000 cycles per second) and emulsifies the lens nucleus so that it may be aspirated from the eye through a small incision; **endocapsular p.** technique in which the emulsification of the nucleus is carried out within the area usually enclosed by the lens capsule, which is opened to allow access to the crystalline lens (*compare* Kelman p.); **endolenticular p.** technique in which the emulsification of the nucleus is carried out entirely within the lens capsule and with the lens nucleus remaining in its natural position within the cortex; **extracapsular p.** technique in which the anterior lens capsule is opened and the nucleus is emulsified through this hole; **intercapsular p.** technique in which the emulsification of the nucleus is carried out through a small slit in the lens capsule; **Kelman p.** original phacoemulsification procedure described by the inventor of phaco, Dr. Charles Kelman, in which the lens nucleus is maneuvered into the anterior chamber and then emulsified; **one-handed p.** general term for techniques of phacoemulsification in which only one instrument (the phaco probe) is used during emulsification of the

nucleus; **two-handed p.** general term for techniques
in which a second instrument is used by the surgeon
to maneuver the lens as it is being emulsified by the
phaco probe.

phacolytic glaucoma: *See* glaucoma.

phakic: State in which the natural lens of the eye is in
place; *compare* aphakic.

phako-: *See* phaco-.

phase: Property of wave energy such that the "peaks"
and "troughs" of many individual waves can coincide
with each other or cancel each other; waves with
peaks and troughs that coincide are said to be in
phase; *see also* coherent light.

phlyctenular keratoconjunctivitis: *See* keratoconjunctivitis.

phlyctenule: Small, fluid-filled blisters that can lead to
ulcerations on the conjunctiva; corneal involvement
can occur; linked to a hypersensitivity to bacterial
products; *see also* phlyctenular keratoconjunctivitis
under keratoconjunctivitis.

phoria: General term for misalignment of the eyes present only when fusion is prevented (by occluding one
eye); it is a latent deviation, usually held in check by
fusion; sometimes called a *heterophoria*; *see also*
esophoria, exophoria, hyperphoria, hypophoria, *and*
orthophoria; *compare* tropia; **horizontal p.** phoria in
the horizontal plane; **vertical p.** phoria in the vertical
plane.

phoropter: Instrument fitted with a number of different
types of lenses that are rotated into place in front of a
test subject's eyes to determine the amount of vision
correction necessary; formerly a brand name of one
such instrument (commonly called a *refractor*) but
now used generically.

photo-: Combining word meaning light.

photoablation: Action of the excimer laser to vaporize
tissue.

photocoagulation: In ophthalmic usage, application of laser light that is absorbed by the pigmented tissues of the eye and converted into heat energy; used to seal blood vessels and for trabeculoplasty; **panretinal p. (PRP)** treatment in which laser is applied to a large area of the retina, as in diabetic retinopathy; *see also* laser.

photodynamic therapy (PDT): Use of low-intensity light (usually from a laser) and photosensitive agents to ablate tissue in a very localized area; in ophthalmology, used to treat ocular tumors, neovascularization, and refractory glaucoma.

photon: Smallest unit (sometimes described as a particle or quantum) of light energy.

photophobia: Excessive sensitivity of the eyes to light.

photopia: Daylight vision in which the rod cells of the retina are suppressed and the cones are the primary light perceiving cells; *compare* mesopia *and* scotopia.

photopsia: Appearance of flashes of light in the field of view attributable to some defect of the retina or optic tract.

photoreceptors: The cells in the retina that transmit nerve impulses when stimulated by light (ie, rod cells and cone cells).

photorefractive keratectomy (PRK): Application of the excimer laser to remove corneal tissue in order to change the surface curvature of the eye and thus correct refractive errors.

phototherapeutic keratectomy (PTK): Application of the excimer laser to remove corneal tissue in order to treat pathology rather than to change any refractive error of the eye.

phototoxicity: Property of bright light such that it damages the retina upon prolonged exposure.

phthisis (pronounced TIE-sis): General term for gradual loss of the bulk and structure of a bodily organ; most commonly in ophthalmic usage referring to *phthisis bulbi*, in which a blind eye shrivels, sometimes necessitating surgical removal.

physiologic astigmatism: *See* astigmatism.

physiologic blind spot or **scotoma:** *See* scotoma.

piggyback intraocular lens: *See* intraocular lens.

pigmentary dispersion syndrome: Condition in which iris pigment is scattered and appears as small deposits on other anterior segment structures but no glaucoma occurs; *compare* pigmentary glaucoma *under* glaucoma.

pigmentary glaucoma: *See* glaucoma.

pinguecula: Abnormal growth of yellowish membrane at the junction of the sclera and cornea that can progress to pterygium.

pinhole (PH): Opaque disk or lens with one or more tiny holes; looking through a pinhole reduces the amount of scattered light, improving any vision decrease due to refractive errors; reduced vision due to pathology is not improved, making pinhole vision an important diagnostic test.

pink eye: Another term for conjunctivitis.

Placido's disk: Disk with concentric circles used to evaluate corneal curvature; *see also* keratoscopy.

plano lens: Lens that has no refracting power; rays of light passing through such a lens (which has no curvature of either surface) continue on their straight-line paths; also, a lens may have one convex or concave surface in combination with one plano surface, in which case it is called *planoconvex* or *planoconcave*, respectively.

platysmal reflex: Constriction of the pupil in response to manipulation of the platysma, a muscle that runs from the neck into the area of the lower jaw.

plica: General anatomic term for a fold of tissue.

plica ciliaris: The small folds of tissue in the ciliary body.

plica lacrimalis: Fold of skin that acts as the valve of the tear gland.

plica semilunaris: Half-moon-shaped fold of tissue formed where the nasal portion of the bulbar conjunctiva joins muscle tissue.

plus: 1. Property of an optical system such that it causes rays of light to converge (eg, a convex lens); 2. in spoken ophthalmic usage, synonym for hyperopia (eg, a "plus 2 diopter patient").

plus lens: Lens that causes rays of light to converge (*see* convex lens *and* cylinder, definition 2); in common ophthalmic usage, the power of the plus sphere lens used to correct farsightedness is often used to describe the degree of hyperopia (thus, a "high plus" or "plus six" patient).

pneumatic retinopexy: *See* retinopexy.

pneumotonometer: *See* tonometer.

polar cataract: *See* cataract.

polarized light: Light that has been altered so that the normally random planes of its transverse wave motions (ie, the plane in which the theoretical "peaks" and "troughs" lie) are aligned along the same pole; polarizing filters are used in various optical instruments and also in some types of sunglasses.

polycarbonate: Lightweight, shatter-resistant polymer used as a spectacle lens material.

polycoria: Condition in which there is more than one pupillary opening in the iris.

polymegethism: In ophthalmic usage, condition in which corneal endothelial cells become irregular in size and shape; note that this spelling is based on authorities' citation of Greek poly ("many") being joined with megethos ("size") rather than megalos ("large").

polymethylmethacrylate (PMMA): Acrylic polymer used in the manufacture of contact lenses ("hard lenses") and intraocular lenses.

polyopia, -sia, -y: General term for visual defect in which one object appears as multiple images; *see also* diplopia.

polypropylene: Flexible polymer used in the manufacture of sutures and some intraocular lens haptics.

posterior capsulotomy: *See* capsulotomy.

posterior chamber (PC): Portion of the eye behind the iris and in front of the crystalline lens-zonule apparatus and ciliary body; it is part of the anterior segment and aqueous is formed here; *compare* anterior chamber; not to be confused with posterior segment.

posterior chamber intraocular lens: *See* intraocular lens.

posterior hyaloid membrane: *See* hyaloid membrane.

posterior pole (of the eye): Imaginary point at the rear surface of the sclera directly opposite the anterior pole of the eye; *compare* anterior pole (of the eye).

posterior pole (of the lens): Point at the very back and center of the crystalline lens; *compare* anterior pole (of the lens).

posterior segment (of the eye): General term describing the structures of the eye lying behind the lens-zonule apparatus and ciliary body; ophthalmic surgery is roughly divided into the categories of anterior segment (cornea, glaucoma, and cataract procedures) and posterior segment (retina and vitreous procedures); not to be confused with posterior chamber; *compare* anterior segment (of the eye).

posterior staphyloma: *See* staphyloma.

posterior subcapsular cataract (PSC): *See* cataract.

posterior synechia (PS): Adhesion of the iris to the lens; *compare* anterior synechia.

posterior toric: Method of stabilizing toric contact lenses by incorporating the toric optics into the posterior surface of the lens, theoretically achieving a shape complementary to that of the cornea, helping to prevent rotation and maintain the orientation of the lens to correct astigmatism in the proper axis; *compare* dynamic stabilization, prism ballast, *and* truncation.

posterior uveitis: Inflammation of the uvea, sometimes simply called uveitis; *compare* anterior uveitis.

posterior vitreous detachment (PVD): Separation of the vitreous body from its normal attachment to the retina, usually following syneresis (ie, degenerative shrinking of the vitreous) but sometimes as a result of trauma; symptoms include flashers and floaters; posterior vitreous detachment sometimes causes retinal breaks, as the posterior vitreous is firmly attached to the retina.

potential acuity: Visual acuity that theoretically could be attained in an eye if all correctable defects (usually referring to opacities of normally clear refractive ocular media) were corrected.

potential acuity meter (PAM): Device that measures potential acuity by projecting an eye chart through any ocular opacities in the ocular media and directly onto the retina; *see also* interferometer.

Prentice's law/rule: Optical formula defining the amount that a ray of light deviates (measured in prism diopters, Δ) from its original straight path when passing through a point at a given distance (measured in centimeters, cm) from the center of a lens of a given power (measured in diopters, D), expressed as $\Delta = D \times cm$.

preretinal membrane: Condition in which a membrane forms between the retina and the vitreous humor in the region of the macula.

presbyope: Individual with presbyopia.

presbyopia: Naturally occurring process of aging whereby changes in ocular tissues result in loss of accommodation and thus near vision, usually first noticeable soon after age 40; these changes are generally considered to be due to increasing rigidity of the crystalline lens and decreasing tone of the ciliary muscle.

pressure: *See* intraocular pressure.

primary: Occurring initially (ie, before a secondary condition, procedure, etc, but not necessarily causing it); *compare* secondary; for entities described as primary, look up entry under main word, such as primary glaucoma *see* glaucoma, etc.

primary deviation: Measurement of a paralytic strabismic deviation in which the normal eye fixates and the fellow eye (with the muscle paralysis) is allowed to deviate; *compare* secondary deviation.

Prince rule: Ruler marked off in inches and/or centimeters, along with dioptric values used to evaluate accommodation; *see also* near point of accommodation *under* accommodation.

principal axis: Another term for optical axis; *see* axis.

prism: 1. General term for a transparent object having at least two flat surfaces at an angle to each other (most commonly a triangle in cross section, the top of which is the apex and the bottom of which is the base) that bends light rays from their original trajectory but in parallel paths; *compare* lens; a prism bends light toward its base, thus when viewed through a prism, an object appears to move toward the prism's apex; prisms are used to measure and/or correct various types of strabismus; **base-down, base-in, base-out,** and **base-up p.** description of the orientation of prisms in front of the eye when measuring strabismus or vergences or when prescribing in a spectacle lens; 2. any component of an optical system that functions as a prism (eg, a concave spectacle lens is thicker around the edges than in the center, bending light more in the periphery of the lens); **induced p.** prismatic effect that occurs when the visual axis of the patient is not aligned with the optic center of a lens.

prism angle: Angle at which the two refracting surfaces of a prism meet.

prism apex: Line formed by the junction of the refracting surfaces of a prism (the top of the triangle).

prism ballast: Method of stabilizing toric contact lenses by thickening the bottom with prism, thereby making the bottom of the lens heavier and/or the top of the lens less resistant to the mechanical action of the lids during blinking, which helps prevent rotation and maintain the orientation of the lens to correct astigmatism in the proper axis; *compare* dynamic stabilization, posterior toric, *and* truncation.

prism bar: Device in which prisms of increasing power are attached together and arranged in a row so that they can be easily moved in front of the eye; **horizontal p.b.** prism bar in which the bases of the prisms are aligned, used for measuring horizontal strabismus; **vertical p.b.** prism bar in which the prisms are arranged apex-to-base-to-apex, used for measuring vertical strabismus.

prism base: Flat, thick surface of a prism opposite the apex.

prism diopter (Δ, PD): Measure of the refracting power of a prism or the prismatic effect of a lens; 1 prism diopter displaces a ray of light 1 centimeter from its original path at a point 1 meter from the prism; *see also* diopter *and* Prentice's law / rule.

progressive addition lens (PAL): Spectacle lens (often referred to as *progressive adds*, *progressives*, or *no-lines*) in which the refractive power increases from the center toward the lower periphery to provide a range of correction from far to near; used in the correction of presbyopia to avoid visible lines on the lens (as seen with traditional bifocal or trifocal lenses).

progressive myopia: *See* myopia.

projection: In ophthalmic usage, process by which objects are mentally connected (via the image on the retina) to various points in space; **anomalous p.** mental connection of an image to a point in space by processes other than those that occur in normal, healthy visual systems; *see also* anomalous retinal correspondence; **erroneous p.** visual defect in which objects are referred to points in space to which they do not actually correspond (ie, the objects seem to be "in the wrong place"); **light p.** *see* light projection.

prolapse: General term for shifting of an anatomic structure out of its normal position and through another structure; *see also* iris prolapse.

proliferative diabetic retinopathy (PDR): *See* diabetic retinopathy.

proliferative vitreoretinopathy (PVR): *See* retinopathy.

proptosis: Protruding eyeball; another term for *exophthalmia*.

protan: Color vision defect involving the red color mechanism and linked to the X chromosome.

protanomaly: Partial impairment of the red color mechanism, resulting in red/green confusion with red appearing duller than normal.

protanopia: Severe lack of the red color mechanism; reds appear black and gray, the orange-yellow-greens all look yellow, blue/green is grayish, and blue looks the same as purple.

provocative test: General term for test in which the examiner attempts to elicit an abnormal response to a stimulus; an example in ophthalmology is provoking high intraocular pressure (eg, when glaucoma is suspected).

pseudo-: Prefix meaning false (eg, pseudostrabismus, where the eyes appear crossed to the observer but on testing are found to be straight).

pseudoaccommodation: Ability to see to some degree at both near and distance when true accommodation is impossible (either because of the onset of presbyopia or in some other circumstance); used to describe range of vision achieved (eg, when a monofocal intraocular lens is implanted in an eye with a low degree of astigmatism).

pseudoexfoliation syndrome: Appearance of flakes (combined with what appears to be iris pigment but is not) on structures of the anterior chamber, including the trabecular meshwork, where they may block aqueous outflow and cause a rise in intraocular pressure; also called *exfoliation syndrome*, with the idea that "true" exfoliation comes from the crystalline lens.

pseudomyopia: Temporary condition of nearsightedness created when spasm of the ciliary muscle puts the eye into a state of accommodation.

pseudophakia: State in which an intraocular lens is present in the eye.

pseudophakic bullous keratopathy: *See* keratopathy.

pseudophakos: Another term for intraocular lens.

pseudopsia: Visual hallucination.

pseudopterygium: *See* pterygium.

pseudoptosis: Apparent drooping of the eyelid that is actually a result of an abnormally narrow fissure; *compare* ptosis.

pseudostrabismus: The eyes appear crossed to the observer but on testing are found to be straight; this optical illusion may be due to epicanthal folds or a large kappa angle.

pseudotumor cerebri: Increase in intracranial pressure on the brain that is *not* due to the presence of a tumor, resulting in ocular symptoms such as blurred and double vision, swelling of the optic nerve head, and strabismus.

pseudo-von Graefe's sign: Failure of the upper eyelid to move downward when the eyeball is turned downward; occurs when nerve fibers serving the eyelid muscles have been damaged and do not heal properly; *compare* von Graefe's sign.

pterygium: Fully attached triangular membrane of fleshy tissue extending from a base in the conjunctiva of the canthus toward and possibly onto the cornea, sometimes arising from a pinguecula; usually caused by excessive exposure of the eye to irritation (eg, dust, wind, and direct sunlight); usually found nasally or temporally; removed surgically if it begins to impinge on the optic axis; **cicatricial p.** or **pseudopterygium** triangular adhesion of the conjunctiva to the cornea resembling pterygium but attached only at its apex; sometimes referred to as a *scar pterygium*.

ptosis: In ophthalmic usage, a drooping of the upper eyelid; **p. adiposa** ptosis caused by the deposit of fatty tissue in the upper eyelid; **false p.** *see* pseudoptosis; **guarding p.** tendency of the lid to droop when the eye has been injured in some way; **Horner's p.** ptosis accompanied by miosis and lack of sweating on one side of the face, caused by a nerve defect; *see also* Horner's syndrome; **levator p.** ptosis caused by a defect of the levator muscle; **morning** or **waking p.** normal drooping of the upper eyelid noted upon waking from sleep.

puncta: Plural of punctum.

punctal occlusion: 1. Method for treating dry eye syndrome by blocking the outflow of tears through the puncta, either temporarily by inserting a punctal plug or permanently by laser cauterization; 2. method of keeping eye drops on the eye and out of systemic circulation by applying pressure to the nasal canthus (with the fingers) after medication has been instilled.

punctal plug: Device that is designed to be inserted into (and later removed from) the punctum in order to treat dry eye by blocking the outflow of tears.

punctum: In ophthalmic usage, one of the openings in the eyelids through which tear fluid drains off of the eye; there is one in the upper (ie, superior p.) and the lower (ie, inferior p.) of each lid, located 2 to 4 mm from the medial canthus; plural: puncta.

pupil (P): Normally circular opening in the center of the iris that controls the amount of light passing through the eye to the retina by opening (dilating) in dim light in a process called *mydriasis* and closing (constricting) in bright light in a process called *miosis*; **fixed p.** pupil in which there is no reaction to light or near; **tonic p.** pupil in which the near reaction of miosis is stronger than the miosis caused by direct light; usually referring to Adie's p.; for a number of other unusual states and abnormal conditions of the pupil that are noteworthy, *see also* Adie's p., Argyll Robertson p., Behr's p., cat's eye p., keyhole p., *and* Marcus Gunn p.

pupillary axis: *See* axis.

pupillary block: Condition in which the iris presses against the structures behind it, blocking the normal flow of aqueous humor into the anterior chamber and resulting in a build-up of intraocular pressure; *see also* iris bombé *and* pupillary block glaucoma *under* glaucoma.

pupillary dilator muscle: Iris muscle encircling the outer edge of the iris and extending into the ciliary body, responsible for dilating the pupil; *compare* pupillary sphincter muscle.

pupillary distance (PD): Measurement of the distance from one pupil's nasal edge to the temporal edge of the pupil of the fellow eye; the idea is to figure the distance between the eyes' visual axes; also called *interpupillary distance (IPD)*.

pupillary margin: Heavily pigmented edge of the iris immediately surrounding the pupil.

pupillary muscle: *See* pupillary dilator muscle *and* pupillary sphincter muscle.

pupillary reflex: Any one of a number of responses of the pupil to a stimulus, usually referring to the reaction of pupil size to varying intensities of light (see details under pupil), but also including **accommodative p.r.** constriction of the pupil in near vision; **consensual p.r.** normal state in which dilation or constriction of one pupil in response to a stimulus is accompanied by a similar response in the pupil of the fellow eye, even if the stimulus is only delivered to one eye; its absence is an indication of the same disorder of the ocular nervous system; **direct p.r.** reaction of pupil size to varying intensities of light in that eye only; **oculosensory p.r.** or **oculopupillary reflex** dilation of the pupils when the surface of the eyeball or eyelids is touched or irritated.

pupillary sphincter muscle: Iris muscle encircling the pupil, responsible for constricting the pupil; *compare* pupillary dilator muscle.

pupillary zone: Area of the iris adjacent to the pupil.

pupillometer: 1. Most commonly, another term for corneal reflection pupillometer; 2. device used to measure pupil size.

pupilloplasty: General term for surgical procedure to alter the appearance or function of the pupil, usually referring to repair of a damaged pupil.

pupilloplegia: Paralysis of the pupil; *see also* fixed pupil *under* pupil.

Purkinje's images: Reflections from the anterior and posterior surfaces of the cornea and crystalline lens, useful in measuring strabismus as well as determining the curvature and relative position of these surfaces (eg, in ophthalmoscopy).

Purkinje's shift: Change in sensitivity of vision from daylight to dark in which the retina becomes more sensitive to the blue-green part of the electromagnetic spectrum; *see also* scotopia.

Q-switched laser: *See* laser.

quadrantanopia, -opsia: Loss of one quarter of the visual field, resulting from some chiasmal or postchiasmal defect such that the visual fields of both eyes are affected; *compare* hemianopia; **crossed binasal q.** quadrantanopia of the lower nasal portion of one visual field and the upper nasal portion of the other visual field; **crossed bitemporal q.** quadrantanopia of the lower temporal portion of one visual field and the upper temporal portion of the other visual field; **heteronymous q.** quadrantanopia affecting different portions of the two visual fields (eg, the upper temporal region of one and the lower nasal region of the other visual field); **homonymous q.** quadrantanopia affecting similar portions of both visual fields (eg, the upper temporal regions of both visual fields); **pie-on-the-floor q.** wedge-shaped quadrantanopia in the lower quadrant; defect occurs in the parietal lobe of the optic radiations; **pie-in-the-sky q.** wedge-shaped quadrantanopia in the upper quadrant and respecting the vertical; defect occurs in the temporal lobe of the optic radiations.

quantum: Fundamental unit of light energy; sometimes called a *particle* or *photon*.

radial keratotomy (RK): Refractive surgical procedure in which corneal incisions are placed radially, like the spokes of a wheel, in order to flatten the cornea and correct nearsightedness; the degree of flattening depends upon the depth (about 90% of the corneal thickness) and number (typically from four to eight) of incisions; *see also* keratotomy.

radiuscope: Instrument for measuring the curvature of contact lenses.

radix: General anatomic term for the "root" of a structure, as in the optic nerve r., which joins the optic nerve to the geniculate body of the brain.

range of motion: In ophthalmology, diagnostic test in which the eyes are rotated to each of the eight cardinal positions in order to evaluate the action(s) of the extraocular muscles; *see also* gaze.

raphe: General anatomic term for the junction line between two halves of a structure; **retinal r.** horizontal line on the temporal side of the macula, dividing superior and inferior fibers of the retinal nerve fiber layer; from the raphe, the nerve fibers follow diverging paths to the optic disk; also called the *horizontal raphe*.

reading vision: Another term for near vision.

recession: In ophthalmology, strabismus surgery in which a muscle is weakened by detaching then reattaching it behind its original insertion point.

rectus muscle: *See* inferior rectus muscle, lateral rectus muscle, medial rectus muscle, *and* superior rectus muscle.

recurrent corneal erosion: *See* corneal erosion.

red-free photography: Photography of the eye using green ("red-free") light, so structures that appear red in white light instead appear black, thereby increasing contrast and enhancing images of blood vessels, inflammation, and hemorrhages.

red reflex: Reflection of light from the retina; appears as a bright red area through the pupil, due to the retina's blood supply and pigmentation; an opacity will cast a shadow or dull the reflex's brightness.

reflection: Property of light such that it bounces back from the surface of an object or from an interface between two substances with different indices of refraction; light rays striking the surface or interface are called *incident* and those bouncing back are called *reflected.*

reflex: 1. Muscle reaction to stimulation; **accommodative r.** the triad of focusing, convergence, and miosis that occurs with near vision; **oculopupillary r.** dilation of the pupils when the globe or lids are irritated; **pupillary r.** *see* pupillary reflex; 2. reflection of light; *see also* red reflex.

refract: 1. To bend light by refraction; *see* refraction, definition 1; 2. to perform a refraction; *see* refraction, definition 2.

refraction: 1. Bending of light as it passes from one transparent media to the next such that light is bent from its normal straight-line course; *see* refractive index; 2. in ophthalmic practice, the act of determining what power lens is needed to correct an ametropia with the intent of generating a prescription for corrective lenses (which may be done only by a licensed professional); *see also* over-refraction; *compare* refractometry; 3. in ophthalmic speech and literature, the power of a lens needed to correct an ametropia is referred to as the refraction of a given individual, leading to informal descriptions such as "the (patient's) refraction was minus 2 diopters;" *see also* manifest refraction.

refractive amblyopia: *See* amblyopia.

refractive error: Another term for ametropia.

refractive index: A comparison between the speed of light traveling through air versus the speed of light as it moves through an optical medium (eg, a lens); the mathematical formula is speed of light in air/speed of light in material = refractive index; a more dense material causes light to pass more slowly through it, and thus has a high refractive index and a higher refracting ability; denser lens materials with a high index of refraction can be fashioned into high-power lenses that are relatively thin.

refractive keratoplasty: Corneal surgery performed to correct refractive error; *see also* keratoplasty *and* refractive surgery.

refractive media: Another term for ocular media; *see also* medium.

refractive surgery: Surgical procedure that has the correction of an ametropia as its primary objective; *see also* clear lensectomy, epikeratophakia, intrastromal corneal ring, keratomileusis, keratophakia, keratoplasty, keratotomy, laser, *and* thermokeratoplasty.

refractometry: Measuring the refractive error of a patient in order to yield information about that refractive error and without writing a prescription for corrective lenses; technical staff may legally perform refractometry but not refractions, as they do not have a license to prescribe; however, licensed personnel may use the refractometric measurement to generate a lens prescription; *compare* refraction, definition 2.

refractor: Instrument containing rotating lenses for the measurement of a patient's refractive error; commonly called a *phoropter*, although that term actually refers to a specific brand of refractor; **automated r. (AR)** computerized instrument that objectively measures a patient's refractive error (and often K readings and pupillary distance as well).

regression: In refractive surgery, phenomenon in which the correction achieved in the immediate postoperative period drifts back toward the original refractive error.

regular astigmatism: *See* astigmatism.

relative afferent pupillary defect (RAPD): Another term for *Marcus Gunn pupil*.

resection: In ophthalmology usage, strabismus surgery in which a muscle is strengthened by shortening and then reattaching it to its original insertion point.

reticule: Pattern of lines or grid, usually a standardized scale, inscribed in the eyepiece of optical instruments to allow the examiner to make quantitative observations of the subject; also called *reticle*.

retina: Transparent, light-sensitive structure lining the inside of the eye; lies between the vitreous body and the choroid; light striking the retina passes through the internal limiting membrane (also known as the *posterior hyaloid face of the vitreous*), the retinal nerve fiber layer, the ganglion cell layer, the inner molecular and inner nuclear layers (which, like the outer molecular and outer nuclear layers just beneath them, are composed of nerve cells and synapses), the external limiting membrane, the bacillary layer (composed of the light-sensitive rod and cone cells), and finally the retinal pigment epithelium (which plays no part in visual sensation but has a key role in retinal nutrition), which is attached to the choroid; *see also* amacrine cells, bipolar cells, fovea, macula, nerve fiber layer, optic disk, *and* ora serrata.

retinal accommodation: Accommodation triggered by the perception of an unfocused image (usually at near) on the retina.

retinal adaptation: Process whereby the retina adjusts to the level of light in the environment, becoming more or less sensitive to light under relatively dark and light conditions, respectively.

retinal apoplexy: Condition in which the central retinal vein is blocked, leading to an impairment of the retina's blood supply and eventual damage.

retinal artery: *See* branch retinal artery *and* central retinal artery.

retinal branch vein occlusion: *See* branch retinal vein occlusion.

retinal central artery occlusion: *See* central retinal artery occlusion.

retinal central vein occlusion: *See* central retinal vein occlusion.

retinal correspondence: Property of vision such that a point on one retina becomes associated (in the brain) with a point on the retina of the fellow eye; if intact, it is known as *normal retinal correspondence (NRC); see* anomalous retinal correspondence *and* harmonious retinal correspondence.

retinal dehiscence: *See* retinal dialysis.

retinal detachment (RD): Condition in which the bacillary layer (rod and cone cells) of the retina is partially or completely separated from the pigment epithelial layer, resulting in a loss of vision in the area that is detached; *see also* giant retinal break *and* retinal tear; **rhegmatogenous r.d.** retinal detachment that begins as a break or tear in the retina, then vitreous seeps in-between the layers; **serous r.d.** detachment in which the layers are forced apart by blood or plasma leaking from retinal blood vessels; **traction r.d.** detachment in which the retina is pulled away from the pigment epithelial layer (eg, as a complication of vitrectomy).

retinal dialysis: Retinal tear in the area of the ora serrata.

retinal dysplasia: General term for abnormal development of retinal tissue.

retinal exudates: Light-colored bodies that appear on the retina in a number of retinal conditions, may be either hard exudates (well-defined, waxy, yellowish bodies that are truly the result of exudation [leakage of substances from retinal tissue]), or soft exudates (which are not exudates at all but rather small areas of the retinal nerve fiber layer that have lost their blood supply and become wispy white zones with no clear borders; also called *cotton-wool spots*); usually appearing in diabetic and other types of retinopathy.

retinal hole: *See* retinal tear.

retinal ischemia: Condition in which the blood supply of the retina is cut off, resulting in tissue damage; *see also* branch retinal artery and vein occlusion, central retinal artery and vein occlusion, *and* retinal exudates.

retinal pigment epithelium (RPE): Dark, posterior-most layer of the retina providing attachment to the choroid as well as functioning in retinal nutrition.

retinal recovery: *See* retinal adaptation.

retinal reflex: *See* red reflex.

retinal rivalry: Blurring of an area of the visual field when different, nonfusable images are presented to corresponding areas of the two retinae as first one image, then the other, is suppressed.

retinal tear: Opening in the retina caused by a pull from the vitreous humor, trauma, or surgical complication; *see also* giant retinal break *and* retinal detachment.

retinal vein: *See* branch retinal vein *and* central retinal vein.

retinitis: General term for inflammation of the retina, often associated with bacteria or fungi and characterized by loss of central vision and cells in the vitreous; may be termed *chorioretinitis* if the choroid is also involved; **actinic r.** retinitis resulting from exposure to ultraviolet radiation; **cytomegalovirus (CMV) r.** opportunistic viral infection (belonging to the Herpes group) of the retina in immunocompromised patients (such as those with AIDS); **exudative r.** retinitis marked by the appearance of retinal exudates; **purulent r.** retinitis caused by infection in the eye; **serous r.** inflammation of the retina characterized by swelling of the macula.

retinitis pigmentosa (RP): Inherited retinal dystrophy in which deposits of melanin pigment appear on the retina, accompanied by atrophy of retinal blood vessels and pallor of the optic disk, eventually leading to loss of vision.

retinoblastoma: Malignant tumor arising from the retinal cells of an embryo and developing in the first few years of life; its hallmark is leukocoria.

retinopathy: General term for abnormal, noninflammatory condition of the retina, often associated with some systemic disorder; **central serous r. (CSR)** sudden edema and swelling of the macula with leakage from blood vessels and central visual impairment and distortion, possibly leading to retinal detachment; **circinate r.** retinopathy marked by the appearance of a circle of white patches around the macula, which can lead to retinal hemorrhaging; **diabetic r.** ocular effects of systemic diabetes mellitus characterized by retinal swelling, multiple small hemorrhages, retinal exudates, and growth of blood vessels into the retina, with progressive loss of vision if left untreated; **hypertensive r.** ocular effects of systemic hypertension, mainly affecting the retinal blood vessels; **proliferative (vitreo-) r.** neovascularization of the retina and vitreous in certain conditions involving the circulatory system, such as diabetes mellitus.

retinopathy of prematurity (ROP): Condition affecting premature infants who are placed in oxygen-enriched environments, occurring less frequently than in the past now that there is increased awareness of risks; marked by neovascularization of the retina, which is followed by retinal hemorrhage, scarring and occasionally detachment, and growth of fibrous tissue into the vitreous humor; the possibility of serious ocular conditions such as glaucoma is increased following retinopathy of prematurity (the advanced stage of which is called *retrolental fibroplasia* [RLF]).

retinopexy: Surgical procedure to repair a retinal detachment, most commonly through injection of air or heavy gas following vitrectomy (pneumatic retinopexy) or sometimes application of extreme cold to the external globe (ie, cryoretinopexy).

retinoschisis: Splitting of the tissue layers of the retina, usually in the periphery (so that central vision is unaffected) and infrequently leading to a detachment.

retinoscope: Hand-held instrument that projects a spot or streak of light that is reflected by the retina; the apparent motion and brightness of the reflected light when the instrument is moved allows the examiner to determine the refractive state of the eye (*see also* neutralization); it is an objective test in that it does not require patient responses.

retinoscopy: Technique of objectively measuring a patient's refractive error using the retinoscope, usually refined via refractometry; **gross r.** the refractive measurement found with the retinoscope, including the power of the working lens; **net r.** the refractive measurement of the eye found with the retinoscope, minus the power of the working lens; this is the patient's actual refractive error.

retinosis: General term for abnormal, noninflammatory condition of the retina.

retinotomy: General term for surgical incision into the retina.

retraction syndrome: Inherited condition marked by very limited ability of the eye to abduct, mildly limited ability to adduct, and partial closure of the eyelids and retraction of the eyeball upon adduction; the eye may shoot up or down in adduction; usually monocular; also called *Duane's retraction syndrome.*

retrobulbar: General term describing the area behind the eye.

retrobulbar anesthesia: Anesthesia administered by injection behind the eye; *compare* peribulbar anesthesia.

retroillumination: Method of viewing an ocular structure by light reflected from another structure (often the retina) lying behind the one to be viewed; usually referring to slit lamp biomicroscopy but can also describe a technique used with the operating microscopes; *see also* indirect illumination.

retrolental: Term describing the area behind the lens.

retrolental fibroplasia (RLF): *See* retinopathy of prematurity.

retroscopic tilt: Undesirable fit of spectacles where the top of the frame front is angled closer to the brow; *compare* pantoscopic tilt.

rhegmatogenous retinal detachment: *See* retinal detachment.

rhodopsin: Light-sensitive retinal pigment found in the rod cells; rhodopsin is synthesized in the dark, obliterated by light, and responsible for dark adaptation; also called *visual purple; see also* scotopia.

rigid gas-permeable (RGP) lens: *See* contact lens.

ring scotoma: *See* scotoma.

river blindness: *See* onchocerciasis.

rod cells: One of two types of light-sensitive cells in the retina; often simply referred to as rods, they function primarily in peripheral and night vision; *compare* cone cells; *see also* rhodopsin *and* scotopia.

rose bengal: Dye used in ophthalmic applications to stain the surface of the eye and detect damaged or dead conjunctival or corneal epithelial cells.

rotatory nystagmus: *See* nystagmus.

Roth's spots: Infectious retinitis in which white areas appear in the optic disk surrounded by areas of hemorrhage.

rubeosis iridis: Abnormal growth of blood vessels into the iris in individuals with diabetes mellitus or following trauma.

saccades: Rapid refixation movements of the eyes from one point of fixation to another in a series of jerky steps, or as an effort to maintain prolonged fixation; *see* also microsaccades.

saccadic fixation: Rapid change of fixation from one point to another in the visual field.

saccadic movement: *See* saccades.

schematic eye: 1. Device used in training for retinoscopy; two telescoping cylinders are used to vary the length of the schematic eye (representing the axial length of a human eye) and auxiliary lenses are placed into the cells of the instrument to simulate astigmatism and other refractive errors; the examiner places trial lenses in front of the auxiliary lens while viewing the schematic eye though the retinoscope; 2. a theoretical eye composed of the average measurements and optical values of ocular structures; the values are used in mathematical computations, but not without inaccuracies; also called *schematic eye of Gullstrand; see* Appendix 3.

Schiøtz tonometer: *See* indentation tonometer *under* tonometer.

Schirmer's test: Test of tear production in which one end of a 5 x 25 mm strip of filter paper is placed into the cul-de-sac of the lower eyelid (about 6 mm temporal of the punctum); the strips are left in place for a 5-minute test time; wetting of the paper at a rate of 2 to 3 mm per minute is considered normal; sometimes referred to as *S.t. number one;* **S.t. number two** same test as above, only the patient is given topical anesthetic prior to inserting the filter strips in order to eliminate tearing caused by irritation of the strips themselves.

Schlemm's canal: Ring-shaped passage in the filtration angle through which aqueous humor drains into the bloodstream.

Schwalbe's line: Border of Descemet's membrane, appearing on gonioscopy as a dark line at the edge of the cornea.

scintillating scotoma: *See* scotoma.

sclera: Commonly called the "white" of the eye; the tough, fibrous tissue that makes up the major outer layer of the eye (lined inside by the choroid and retina); the optic nerve passes through it posteriorly at the lamina cribrosa, and anteriorly it joins with the clear cornea at the limbus; **blue s.** appearance of a thin sclera when pigment and blood from underlying tissue (the choroid) gives it a bluish tint.

scleral buckle (SB): Elastic band placed around the globe as part of a procedure to repair a retinal detachment.

scleral buckling procedure: General term for surgical techniques to repair retinal detachment in which a device (such as an elastic band) is used to indent the sclera in the region of the detachment, bringing the pigment epithelium layer back into contact with the bacillary layer of the retina.

scleral canal: *See* Schlemm's canal.

scleral conjunctiva: *See* bulbar *under* conjunctiva.

scleral foramen: Another term for lamina cribrosa.

scleral lens: Large-diameter contact lens that covers the cornea and extends over the conjunctiva and onto the sclera used in orthokeratology and treatment of certain conditions of the external ocular tissues; *compare* semiscleral lens; *see also* contact lens.

scleral show: Excessive exposure of the sclera due to abnormally wide opening of the eyelids.

scleral spur: Band of scleral fibers in the anterior chamber, located between Schlemm's canal and the ciliary body, serving as part of the anchor tissue for the ciliary body and iris.

scleral sulcus: Area where the tissues of the cornea insert into the similarly fibrous tissues of the sclera.

scleral trabeculae: Another term for trabecular meshwork.

sclerectasia, -asis: Stretching of the sclera caused by chronic elevated intraocular pressure in early life.

sclerectomy: General term for surgical removal of scleral tissue.

scleritis: Inflammation of the sclera; **anterior s.** scleritis affecting the front, visible part of the sclera; **necrotizing s.** slowly progressive degeneration of the sclera to the point of perforation, often associated with rheumatoid arthritis; also called *scleromalacia perforans*; **posterior s.** scleritis affecting the back, nonvisible portion of the sclera and Tenon's capsule.

sclerocorneal: Of or related to the sclera and cornea together.

scleromalacia: Condition marked by the thinning and softening of the sclera.

scleromalacia perforans: Another term for *necrotizing scleritis; see* scleritis.

scleronyxis: Surgical procedure involving a puncturing of the sclera.

scleroplasty: General term for surgical procedure on the sclera.

sclerostomy: General term for the surgical creation of an opening in the sclera, most commonly in an attempt to allow drainage of aqueous from the anterior chamber in the treatment of glaucoma.

sclerotic scatter: In slit lamp biomicroscopy, method of shining the light onto the corneal limbus from an angle, creating a bright ring around the cornea; this light is refracted throughout corneal tissue to provide a view of its structure, especially the general pattern of any opacities.

sclerotomy: General term for an incision into the sclera.

scoto-: Combining word meaning dark.

scotoma: Area within the borders of the visual field in which vision is impaired or absent, attributable to dysfunction of the retina or optic nerve; plural: scotomata; *see also* hemianopia *and* quadrantanopia (both of which are contractions of the field rather than scotomata); **absolute s.** area within the visual field where there is no response to any stimuli (of that particular perimeter); **annular s.** ring-shaped scotoma, usually centered around the fixation point; **arcuate s.** nerve fiber bundle defect that curves in an arc-like shape; also called *scimitar scotoma*; **Bjerrum's s.** scotoma extending from the physiologic blind spot (if it progresses it becomes an arcuate scotoma); **central s.** scotoma in the center of the visual field with corresponding impairment of macular function; **centrocecal s.** egg-shaped scotoma extending from the physiologic scotoma to the fixation point; **comet s.** another term for arcuate s.; **false s.** area of impairment in the visual field that is not attributable to dysfunction of the retina (eg, scotoma caused by a small undiagnosed cataract); **junction s.** scotoma arising from a defect in the optic chiasm (junction of the two optic nerves); **motile s.** type of false scotoma in which opaque material (eg, cells) floating through the vitreous results in the appearance of dark areas within the visual field that shift with the passing of time; **negative s.** scotoma that is dark and devoid of light perception; **paracentral s.** near-central scotoma attributable to an area of dysfunction close to the macula; **pericecal** or **peripapillary s.** scotoma occurring around the physiologic blind spot related to nerve fiber dysfunction near the disk; **peripheral s.** scotoma that is located well away from the fixation point; **physiologic s.** another term for blind spot; **positive s.** scotoma that is bright, often scintillating; **relative s.** area within an isopter where the retina does not respond to the target used to map the isopter; **ring s.** another term for annular s.; **scimi-**

tar s. another term for arcuate s.; **scintillating s.** scotoma with a jagged outline surrounded by bright flashes, often reported to precede attacks of migraine; **Seidel's s.** arcuate defect that has extended from a Bjerrum's scotoma at the physiologic blind spot and curves around the central field.

scotopia: Night vision in which the rod cells of the retina are sensitized with the pigment rhodopsin in the process of dark (scotopic) adaptation; *compare* nyctalopia *and* photopia; *see also* Purkinje's shift.

secondary: Occurring sequentially after some preexisting condition, procedure, etc, but not necessarily as a result of it; *compare* primary; for conditions described as secondary, look up entry under main word, such as secondary cataract *see* cataract, secondary glaucoma *see* glaucoma, etc; follow same approach for devices and procedures, such as secondary IOL *see* intraocular lens, etc.

secondary deviation: The amount of deviation that occurs in paralytic strabismus when the eye that normally does not fixate is forced to do so; the secondary deviation is always larger than the primary deviation; *compare* primary deviation.

sector iridectomy: *See* sector i. *under* iridectomy.

segment: 1. In general ophthalmology, referring to the anterior or posterior of the eye, with the crystalline lens being the dividing line; **anterior s.** front portion of the eye from (and including) the crystalline lens forward; comprised of both anterior and posterior chambers; **posterior s.** rear portion of the eye from behind the crystalline lens and back; 2. in opticianry, term used to describe the near vision optical element(s) placed into a portion of a corrective bifocal or trifocal lens; *see also* add.

segment height: Millimeter measurement indicating the placement of any multifocal add(s) to a spectacle lens; measured from the deepest part of the eyewire.

Seidel's scotoma: *See* scotoma.

Seidel's sign: Leakage of aqueous humor from the anterior chamber onto the external surface of the eye made visible with the use of fluorescein dye.

semilunar fold: Flap of conjunctiva normally found in the medial canthus next to the caruncle.

semiscleral lens: Contact lens that covers the cornea and extends slightly past the limbus; modern soft lenses are of this type; *compare* scleral lens.

senile: General term meaning occurring in old age; *compare* congenital, infantile, *and* juvenile.

senile cataract: *See* cataract.

senile ectropion: Ectropion occurring in elderly individuals due to the loss of elasticity of the tissues of the eyelid.

senile macular degeneration (SMD): *See* macular degeneration (age-related).

sensory fusion: *See* fusion.

sensory retina: All layers of the retina involved in the perception of light (ie, all layers except the retinal pigment epithelium); *see also* retina.

Sherrington's law of reciprocal innervation: General principle of physiology, also applicable to the extraocular muscles, that every stimulus inducing a muscle to contract is accompanied by an equal stimulus for the antagonistic muscle (ie, the one with the opposite effect) to relax.

siderosis: General term for condition in which deposits of iron appear in bodily tissues.

siderosis bulbi: Siderosis within the eye.

siderosis conjunctivae: Deposits of iron in the conjunctiva, usually from a foreign body.

sign: Objective finding associated with a disorder that can be perceived or detected by the examiner; *compare* symptom.

silicone contact lens: *See* soft contact lens *under* contact lens.

silicone IOL: *See* intraocular lens.

silicone oil: Heavy fluid used in surgery to repair retinal detachment; *see also* gas-fluid exchange.

sine-wave grating: *See* contrast sensitivity test.

sinistro-: Prefix describing processes or structures occurring or appearing toward the left; in ophthalmic usage, part of the phrase oculus sinister (OS), meaning the left eye; *compare* dextro-.

Sjögren's syndrome: Systemic disorder with symptoms including severe dry eye, dry mouth, and connective tissue disease (most commonly rheumatoid arthritis); *see also* ortho-ophthalmopathy.

skew deviation: *See* deviation.

skiascopy: Another term for retinoscopy.

slab-off lens: Multifocal lens in which a portion of the lower near-vision segment is ground away (thus the term *slab-off*) in such a way as to shift the optical center of that segment closer to the optical center of the upper distance vision part of the lens; this is done to reduce the vertical imbalance (thus eliminating double vision and discomfort) present at near when there is a large difference in refractive error between the two eyes.

slit lamp: Microscope with a light source that projects a beam of light onto the eye, usually as a narrow vertical beam (thus, the term *slit*, but with other beam shapes possible), allowing an examiner to view ocular structures under varying magnifications and illuminations.

slit lamp biomicroscopy: Examination of a patient using the slit lamp.

Sloan letters or **optotypes:** Eye chart or card using block capital letters C, D, H, K, N, O, R, S, V, and Z.

Snell's law: Optical formula defining the index of refraction of a substance as the sine of the angle of incidence divided by the sine of the angle of refraction.

Snellen's acuity: Measurement of visual acuity based upon standard sizes of letters visible to the "normal" eye at specified distances; the test type incorporated into Snellen's vision test target is the most commonly used eye chart in the United States; its standard testing distance of 20 feet gives us the familiar system of measuring distance visual acuity against a reference value of 20/20.

Soemmering's ring: Ring-shaped collection of crystalline lens material left after cataract extraction, which sometimes opacifies.

soft contact lens (SCL): *See* contact lens.

soft exudates: *See* retinal exudates.

soft IOL: *See* intraocular lens (foldable).

spectacles: Eyeglasses; **aphakic s.** eyeglasses prescribed to correct vision after removal of a cataractous crystalline lens, usually requiring very thick plus lenses; **half-eye s.** small spectacles, often with a flat top, made to wear farther down on the nose than normal so that one may look through them when gazing down for near work and over them when looking straight ahead at a distance.

spectrum: *See* electromagnetic spectrum.

specular microscopy: Technique for viewing the corneal endothelium; used to assess the health of the cornea, particularly prior to ophthalmic surgery.

speculum: General term for an instrument that facilitates the observation of some part of the body by holding open an orifice; in ophthalmic usage, a lid speculum refers to a device placed between the upper and lower lids to hold them open.

sphenoid bone: One of the bones of the orbit.

sphenoid fissure: The superior orbital fissure; *see* orbital fissure.

sphere (sph): 1. In optics, a lens that refracts all incoming light to a single focal point; 2. in refraction, the component of refractive error that can be corrected with a spherical lens (myopia or hyperopia); *compare* cylinder.

spherical aberration: Uneven refraction of light through the periphery of a lens.

spherical equivalent (Deq SE): 1. Representation of the refractive power of a toric lens defined as the spherical power plus one half the cylinder power; 2. similar calculation performed on the components of a spectacle prescription to describe the overall refractive error of an eye.

spherical lens: Lens that refracts all incoming light to a single focal point; *compare* aspheric.

spherocylindrical lens: A lens combining spherical (for hyperopia or myopia) and astigmatic (cylindrical) correction; *see also* toric lens.

sphincter: General anatomic term for a circular muscle; in ophthalmic usage, referring to the pupillary sphincter.

sphincterotomy: In ophthalmic usage, an incision into the pupillary sphincter, usually performed when a small pupil makes intraocular surgery difficult.

spindle cells: Another term for Krukenberg's spindles.

spiral of Tillaux: Configuration of the insertion-to-limbus distances of the extraocular muscles such that the distances decrease as you go around the limbus; on the right eye, beginning superiorly and moving counterclockwise, these measurements are superior oblique (7.7 mm), lateral rectus (7.0 mm), inferior rectus (6.5 mm), and medial rectus (5.5 mm).

spot retinoscope: Retinoscope that projects a round light; *see also* retinoscope.

squint: Largely out-of-date term for strabismus.

squint angle: *See* angle of deviation.

staining: *See* corneal staining.

staphyloma: Localized thinning of the sclera so that it bulges, often associated with high myopia; it appears dark because the choroid pushes into the bulging area; rarely referring to a thinned, bulging area of the cornea; **anterior s.** scleral staphyloma in the area of the ciliary body; **equatorial s.** scleral staphyloma occurring midway between the anterior and posterior poles of the eye, usually where the vortex veins exit the globe; **posterior s.** scleral staphyloma in the posterior segment, usually at the optic nerve head.

static perimetry: *See* perimetry.

steep: In ophthalmic usage, describing the surface curvature of a lens or ocular medium that imparts the greatest refractive power; *compare* flat.

steep axis: In a toric lens or spherocylindrical ocular medium (usually the cornea), the most curved axis that hence has the most refracting power; the cylinder axis of astigmatism as measured on refractometry using plus cylinder is parallel to this steep axis (in minus cylinder it is perpendicular to it).

steepening: In refractive surgery, increasing the curvature of the cornea to correct hyperopia; *compare* flattening.

step: *See* nasal step.

stereopsis: Three-dimensional vision possible only when binocular vision and fusion are present; *see also* binocular vision *and* fusion; *compare* depth perception.

steroids: Another term for corticosteroids.

stigmatic lens: Lens that brings light from a point source into a point of focus.

stigmatoscopy: Technique for determining the refractive state of the eye by having the test subject view a pinpoint of light and report its appearance.

strabismus: Misalignment of the visual axes of the eyes (ie, the eyes are not straight); commonly called *crossed eyes; see also* angle of deviation, primary deviation, *and* secondary deviation; **absolute s.** strabismus present under all conditions and at all fixation distances; **accommodative s.** strabismus (usually convergent) that occurs upon accommodation or attempted accommodation; *see also* esotropia; **alternating s.** strabismus in which either eye can maintain fixation (also called *bilateral* or *binocular s.*); **anatomic s.** strabismus resulting from malformation of the structure of the eye, ocular muscles, or orbit; **comitant** or **concomitant s.** strabismus in which the angle of deviation is the same for all directions of gaze regardless of which eye is fixating; *compare* incomitant s.; **constant s.** *see* absolute s.; **convergent s.** strabismus in which the deviation is inward/nasal/medial (also called *esotropia* or *internal strabismus*); **cyclic s.** strabismus that occurs and disappears at regular intervals of time; **divergent s.** strabismus in which the deviation is outward/temporal/lateral (also called *exotropia* or *external strabismus*); **dynamic s.** muscular imbalance that tends to make the eye deviate but is usually overcome in normal binocular vision; **horizontal s.** strabismus in which the misalignment is to the left or right; *compare* vertical s.; **incomitant s.** paralytic strabismus in which the angle of deviation varies with the direction of gaze, fixating eye, or fixation distance; *compare* comitant s.; **intermittent s.** strabismus that is not present at all times; **kinetic s.** strabismus resulting from spasm of the extraocular muscles; **latent s.** misalignment of the eye that occurs only when one eye is deprived of fusional stimulus; *see* phoria; **manifest s.** strabismus that is not latent; *see* tropia; **mechanical s.** strabismus resulting from some anatomic pull upon or displacement of the eye or extraocular muscles; **microstrabismus** strabismus of such a small degree that it is only noted upon close examination; **muscular s.** strabismus resulting from some imbalance of the extraocular muscles; **monolateral** or **monocular s.** another term for unilateral s.; **noncomitant** or **nonconcomitant s.** another term for incomitant s.; **paralytic s.** strabismus resulting from paralysis of one or more extraocular muscles; **periodic** or **relative s.** strabismus that occurs only at certain directions of gaze or fixation distances; **spasmodic** or **spastic s.** strabismus resulting from spasm of one or more extraocular muscles; **suppressed s.** another term for latent s.; **unilateral s.** strabismus in which one eye deviates while the fellow eye achieves normal fixation; **vertical s.** strabismus in which the deviation is a turning up or down; *compare* horizontal s.

strabotomy: Surgical procedure to correct strabismus by cutting an extraocular muscle.

streak retinoscope: Retinoscope that projects a linear light reflex; *see also* retinoscopy.

striae: General medical term for the appearance of lines or streaks in tissue; **corneal s.** fine, whitish lines in the corneal stroma resulting from edema; **retinal s.** lines in the retina, usually originating from a visible point of pathology.

stroma: General anatomic term for the main structural element of a tissue or organ; **corneal s.** central layer of fibrous corneal tissue lying between Bowman's and Descemet's membranes; **iris s.** connective tissue to which the sphincter muscles, nerves, and pigment of the iris adhere.

Sturm's interval: In astigmatism, the area between the point focus of the spherical component and the linear focus of the astigmatic component; light rays within this interval form a cone shape known as the *conoid of Sturm.*

sty: Another term for external hordeolum.

subcapsular cataract: *See* cataract.

subchoroidal hemorrhage: Bleeding between the retina and choroid, leading to retinal detachment if left untreated (sometimes called *suprachoroidal hemorrhage*).

subconjunctival hemorrhage (SCH): Bleeding between the conjunctiva and sclera, dramatic in appearance (initially a blood-red patch on the surface of the eye) but usually posing no threat to eye or sight and resolving without treatment.

subduction: General term for downward motion; in ophthalmic usage, downward movement of the eye.

subjective: Method of testing that relies on the patient's responses (eg, refractometry, Maddox rod, stereo testing); *compare* objective.

subluxation: General term for dislocation, as in a subluxated lens.

substantia propria corneae and **sclerae:** Stroma of the cornea and sclera, respectively.

sulcus: General anatomic term describing a grooved or depressed area; *see also* ciliary sulcus *and* scleral sulcus.

sulfonamide: Any sulfa-containing drug used as an antibacterial.

sulfur hexafluoride (SF$_6$): Heavy gas used in surgery to repair retinal detachment.

sunrise and **sunset syndromes:** Dislocation of an intraocular lens upward or downward, respectively, behind the pupil.

supercilium: Proper term for the eyebrow.

superficial punctate keratitis (SPK): *See* keratitis.

superior oblique muscle (SO): Extraocular muscle lying across the top of the eye responsible for depressing, abducting, and intorting the eye.

superior rectus muscle (SR): Extraocular muscle lying across the top of the eye responsible for elevating, adducting, and intorting the eye.

suppression: Action of the brain to ignore the image from one eye during binocular vision as a result of anisometropia, deviation, or other visual disturbance.

suprachoroid: The outer layer of the choroid and ciliary body consisting primarily of connective, avascular tissue.

supraduction: In ophthalmic usage, upward turning of one eye; also called *sursumduction* and *elevation*.

supraorbital: At the top of or above the bony eye socket.

supraversion: In ophthalmic usage, upward turning of both eyes; also called *sursumversion* and *elevation*.

surgical reversal of presbyopia (SRP): Four plastic segments are inserted into the sclera in the area of the ciliary body in order to create more tension on the zonules; *compare* laser reversal of presbyopia.

sursumduction: Another term for supraduction.

sursumversion: Another term for supraversion.

swinging flashlight test: Pupil test in which the light source is moved rapidly from one eye to the other while evaluating pupillary reaction; *see also* Marcus Gunn pupil.

symblepharon: Condition in which the conjunctiva of the eyelid adheres to the bulbar conjunctiva.

sympathetic amaurosis: *See* amaurosis.

sympathetic nervous system: Division of the autonomic nervous system that diverts energy to the muscles for "fight or flight;" in the eye, this system causes pupil dilation; *see also* adrenergic *and* epinephrine; *compare* parasympathetic nervous system.

sympathetic ophthalmia (SO): Condition in which trauma or intraocular foreign body leading to uveitis in one eye is followed by uveitis in the other uninjured eye a few weeks later; in some cases of trauma, a severely injured eye will be removed to prevent this complication; although rare, it causes a loss of sight in both eyes.

sympatholytic: Substance that blocks the sympathetic system, thus causing a parasympathetic response; beta-blockers, used to treat glaucoma, are sympatholytic drugs; *compare* parasympatholytic.

sympathomimetic: Substance that causes a sympathetic-like response; also called *adrenergic*; phenylephrine (a mydriatic) is a sympathomimetic drug; *compare* parasympathomimetic.

symptom: Subjective indication or perception of a disorder as experienced and related by the patient; may or may not be objectively apparent to the examiner (eg, an examiner and patient can both see redness, but only the patient can feel pain); *compare* sign.

synapse: A gap between the axon of one nerve cell and the dendrite of the next; impulses cross the synapse via neurotransmitters; *see also* axon, dendrite, *and* neurotransmitter.

syncanthus: Adhesion of the tissues of the eye to structures of the orbit.

synchysis: Condition in which the vitreous humor loses its normal consistency and liquifies; **s. scintillans** formation of sparkling crystals within the liquefied vitreous humor, related to ocular degenerative disease.

synechia: General term for fibrous adhesion of organs or tissues; plural: synechiae; *see also* anterior synechiae.

synechialysis: Surgical breaking of synechiae.

syneresis: In ophthalmic usage, degenerative shrinking of the vitreous body as a result of aging, often resulting in vitreous detachment.

synoptophore: Table-top instrument used in measuring strabismus, testing retinal correspondence, and orthoptic training.

tangent screen: A method of manual perimetry using a large black felt screen to find scotomata and map isopter borders in the central 30 degrees of the visual field; targets of varying sizes and colors are presented by the examiner, and the patient indicates when they are seen or not seen.

tangential illumination: In slit lamp biomicroscopy, method of viewing surfaces of ocular structures (especially their texture) by shining light at an oblique angle across the surface of the structure.

tarsal: Of or like the tarsus.

tarsal angle: Another term for canthus.

tarsal glands: Another term for meibomian glands.

tarsal muscle: One of the muscles that acts to open the eyelids, either upper (superior tarsal muscle, also called *Müller's muscle*) or lower (inferior tarsal muscle).

tarsal plate: *See* tarsus.

tarsorrhaphy: General term for surgical procedures in which the upper and lower eyelids are sutured together.

tarsus: "Plate" of connective tissue that serves as the underlying structure of the eyelids, either upper (superior tarsus) or lower (inferior tarsus); plural: tarsi.

tear break-up time: Another term for break-up time.

tear duct, gland, etc: *See* lacrimal apparatus.

tear film: The natural fluid covering of the surface of the eye, composed primarily of three strata: an inner layer of mucin (produced in the conjunctival goblet cells), a middle watery layer (produced in the lacrimal glands, which also produce various important tear proteins like lactoferrin), and an outer layer of oily lipid secretions (produced in the meibomian glands); contact lenses "ride" upon the tear film, which is constantly refreshed by the various glands mentioned above and continuously drains through the puncta and the nasolacrimal ducts into the nasal sinuses.

telescope: 1. General term for an optical device consisting of an objective (either a convex lens or concave mirror) and an ocular (a concave or convex lens) to enlarge and focus the image of a distant object; **Galilean t.** telescope in which the objective is a convex lens and the ocular is a concave lens, producing an erect image; 2. low-vision aid that employs telescopic optics to magnify a relatively narrow field of view.

temple: In opticianry, part of the spectacle frame that attaches to the frame front, rests against the head, and usually extends over the ear; *see also* frame front.

temporal: General anatomic directional term meaning toward the side (ie, temple) of the head; *see also* lateral; *compare* medial *and* nasal.

temporal canthus: Another term for lateral canthus.

tenectomy: Surgical procedure in which a tendon is cut and removed (not to be confused with tenonectomy).

Tenon's capsule, membrane, or **sac:** Thin, outermost membrane enclosing the eye from the limbus back to the optic nerve, including some muscle tendons; also called *fascia bulbi*.

tenonectomy: Surgical removal of a portion of Tenon's capsule.

tenonotomy: Surgical procedure in which an incision is made into Tenon's capsule.

tenotomy: Surgical procedure in which a tendon is cut (not to be confused with tenonotomy).

thermokeratoplasty (TK): Refractive surgical procedure to correct farsightedness in which heat is applied to the sclera at points around the cornea to shrink scleral tissue, thus steepening the cornea.

thimerosal: Mercuric preservative/antiseptic used in some topical ophthalmic medications and contact lens care solutions; currently not much in use because of frequent allergic responses.

thyroid eye disease: Set of ocular dysfunctions associated with Graves' disease.

tonic pupil: Generally another term for Adie's pupil; *see* pupil.

Tono-Pen: *See* tonometer.

tonography: A method of determining aqueous outflow by measuring changes in intraocular pressure constantly over a period of time as a weight is applied to the eye.

tonometer: Instrument that measures intraocular pressure; **air-puff t.** another term for pneumotonometer; **applanation t. (A, Ap,** or **AT)** tonometer that measures intraocular pressure by quantifying the resistance of the eye to flattening; the tonometer tip flattens the cornea a specific amount and measures the pressure needed to do so (also called *applanometer*); **Goldmann t.** classic applanation tonometer design employing a split prism to create mires that indicate the endpoint of the reading; often attached to the slit lamp; **indentation t.** tonometer that measures intraocular pressure by quantifying the degree to which the eye can be indented by a given weight (eg, the Schiøtz tonometer); **MacKay-Marg electronic t.** tonometer that measures intraocular pressure using principles of both applanation and indentation; gives a printout of every corneal contact; **noncontact t. (NCT)** another term for pneumotonometer; **Perkins t.** hand-held Goldmann tonometer; **pneumotonometer** type of noncontact tonometer that uses a puff of air to measure intraocular pressure; **Tono-Pen t.** (Intermedics Intraocular, Pasadena, Calif) brand name of handheld, portable tonometer that gives an electronic readout of intraocular pressure when placed against the cornea.

tonometry: The act of measuring intraocular pressure using a tonometer; **digital t.** method of measuring approximate intraocular pressure by pressing against the eye with a finger.

topography: *See* corneal topography.

toric lens: Spectacle or contact lens having spherical and cylindrical components of curvature, prescribed to correct vision in an eye with astigmatism plus myopia or hyperopia; *see also* aspheric *and* spherocylindrical lens; *compare* spherical lens.

torsion: Rotational ocular movement along the long axis of the eye.

trabecular meshwork (TM): In ophthalmic usage, the porous tissues at the junction of the ciliary body and sclera through which aqueous humor drains from the anterior chamber of the eye.

trabeculectomy: General term for a surgical procedure in which tissue is removed from the trabecular meshwork most often to treat glaucoma by allowing aqueous humor to drain more easily from the eye.

trabeculoplasty: General term for surgical procedures (most commonly describing laser surgical procedures such as argon laser trabeculoplasty [ALT]) that attempt to modify the structure of the trabecular meshwork and increase the outflow of aqueous humor in eyes with glaucoma; *see also* laser.

trabeculotomy: General term for a surgical procedure involving an incision into the trabecular meshwork.

trachoma: Inflammation of the cornea and conjunctiva caused by infection with Chlamydia organisms, leading to severe scarring (especially under the lids) and blindness if not treated; the leading cause of blindness worldwide, especially in third-world countries; **t. inclusion conjunctivitis (TRIC)** reference name given to the intracellular parasite that causes trachoma.

traction retinal detachment: *See* retinal detachment.

transillumination: In slit lamp biomicroscopy, evaluation of an ocular structure (often the lens and iris) by noting how light passes through it.

transposition: Mathematical manipulation of a glasses or contact lens prescription in order to change from plus cylinder form to minus or vice versa; the procedure is as follows: algebraically add the spherical and cylindrical powers (this becomes the new spherical power), change the sign of the original cylinder (without changing its value), and rotate the axis by 90 degrees (if the original axis is 90 or less, add 90; if the original axis is over 90 degrees, subtract 90).

traumatic cataract: *See* cataract.

trephine: Surgical instrument consisting of an open cylinder with a sharp end for cutting a circular incision, typically used in ophthalmic surgery to make an incision around the edge of the cornea so it can be removed; *see also* penetrating keratoplasty.

trial frame: Specially designed, adjustable spectacle frame in which various trial lenses can be placed to measure a refractive error.

trial lens: 1. Loose spectacle lenses used in a trial frame; 2. contact lens used to check the fit before prescribing final lenses.

trichiasis: Condition in which individual lashes are turned inward toward the globe and irritate ocular surface tissues.

trichromatism: Condition in which all three visual pigments are present; *see also* chlorolabe, cyanolabe, *and* erythrolabe; *compare* achromatism *and* monochromatism; **anomalous t.** condition in which all three visual pigments are present but one is deficient, causing a defect in color vision.

trifocal lens: Spectacle lens with three different segments that focus at near, medium, and far distances; *compare* bifocal lens.

tritan: Color vision defect involving the blue color mechanism.

tritanomaly: Color vision defect in which the blue pigment is partially deficient, causing blue/green and yellow/green confusion; violets are perceived normally.

tritanopsia: Severe lack of the blue color mechanism; reds and greens are normal, but yellow-green through purple (including blue) appear white and gray.

trochlea: Ring of cartilaginous tissue attached to the frontal bone through which the tendon of the superior oblique muscle passes.

trochlear nerve (CR IV): The fourth cranial nerve, a motor nerve that supplies the superior oblique muscle.

tropia: Constant (manifest) misalignment of the eyes in which they fail to fixate on the same object; commonly called *crossed eyes*; also called *heterotropia*; *see also* esotropia, exotropia, *and* strabismus; *compare* phoria; **horizontal t.** tropia in which the eyes deviate in or out (ie, left or right); **vertical t.** tropia in which the eyes deviate up or down.

troposcope: Another term for amblyoscope.

truncation: Method of stabilizing toric contact lenses by flattening one edge of the lens (usually the inferior) so that it is no longer round, thereby creating a linear edge that rests against the lid margin; truncation is employed to help prevent rotation and maintain the orientation of toric contact lenses in the proper axis; *compare* dynamic stabilization, posterior toric, *and* prism ballast.

tunnel field: Nonphysiologic visual field loss in which the patient's "tunnel vision" does not expand with increased distance, as does true tunnel vision; usually associated with hysteria or malingering.

tunnel vision: True visual field defect in which only a small central portion of the visual field remains functional.

20/20: Considered to be "normal" vision, the denominator stands for the standard 20-foot test distance used in measuring distant visual acuity; the numerator represents the smallest line of test objects accurately identified by the patient from 20 feet away; 20/40 would mean that the patient could identify figures from 20 feet that the "normal" person could identify from 40 feet away (thus, the larger the numerator, the poorer the vision).

typoscope: Low-vision aid consisting of a rectangle of dark, nonreflective material with a narrow horizontal slit through which type can be read, thereby minimizing glare from the page and isolating the words being read.

UGH syndrome: Abbreviation for combination of uveitis, glaucoma, and hyphema; inflammatory condition of internal ocular structures occurring as a complication of intraocular lens implantation.

ultrasonography: Imaging internal structures via the use of ultrasound techniques.

ultrasound: Imaging technique that uses sound waves to produce an image; in ophthalmology, used to measure the axial length of the eye as well as to visualize the eye's inner structures; *see* A-scan *and* B-scan.

ultraviolet (UV): Portion of the electromagnetic spectrum with short wavelengths, not visible to the human eye; ultraviolet radiation causes sunburn and tanning and has been implicated in certain ocular conditions, notably corneal burns and cataract formation.

ultraviolet A (UVA) and B (UVB): The two bands of ultraviolet radiation.

ultraviolet blocker: Substance incorporated into spectacle, contact, and intraocular lenses to shield the eye from the ultraviolet component of sunlight.

uncorrected visual acuity (UCVA, VA$_{sc}$): Visual acuity measured without corrective lenses in place; *compare* best corrected visual acuity.

undercorrection: State in which the power of corrective lenses or the effect of refractive surgery is insufficient to achieve the best visual acuity; *compare* overcorrection.

unilateral: General anatomic term describing a structure or process appearing or occurring on only one side; in ophthalmic usage, referring to a single eye; *see also* monocular; *compare* bilateral.

uniocular: 1. Another term for monocular; 2. another term for unilateral.

uvea: The tissues of the eye that are heavily pigmented and consist primarily of blood vessels: the choroid, ciliary body, and iris (considered as a whole system).

uveitis: Inflammation of all or part of the uvea; **anterior u.** uveitis involving only the iris and/or ciliary body; *see also* iridocyclitis *and* iritis; **phacolytic u.** uveitis resulting from degeneration and leakage of lens tissue; **posterior u.** uveitis involving only the choroid, often referred to simply as uveitis, creating confusion as to what is meant.

V pattern: *See* esotropia and exotropia.

Van Lint block: Injection of anesthetic agents to achieve akinesia (ie, prevention of movement) of the eyelids.

vault: *See* apical clearance, definition 1.

vergence: 1. In optics, the gathering together or spreading apart of parallel light rays, either naturally or as a result of passing through a lens; *see also* convergence *and* divergence; 2. in ophthalmic usage, motion of the eyes toward or away from one another; *see also* convergence *and* divergence; *compare* duction.

verification: Measuring the parameters of a contact lens, spectacle lens, or pair of spectacles to be sure that the items match what was ordered prior to dispensing to the patient.

vernal conjunctivitis: *See* conjunctivitis.

version: Coordinated movement of both eyes in the same direction.

vertex distance: Distance along the line of sight from the cornea to the back surface of a spectacle lens.

vertex power: Focusing power of a spectacle lens measured from either of its surfaces; **back v.p.** portion of the total refractive power imparted by the posterior surface of a lens; **front v.p.** portion of the total refractive power imparted by the anterior surface of a lens.

videokeratography: Another term for corneal topography.

viscodissection: Surgical technique in which a viscoelastic substance is injected between tissues (commonly the tissues surrounding the lens nucleus) in order to separate them and facilitate subsequent manipulation; *compare* hydrodissection.

viscoelastic material: Any one of a number of thick gels manufactured for use in ophthalmic surgery, injected into the eye to help maintain the shape of ocular structures and as a lubricant/coating to minimize trauma from surgical instruments and implants; currently used viscoelastic materials include chondroitin sulfate, hyaluronic acid, and methylcellulose (used individually or in combination and marketed under several brand names).

vision: Action of the eyes, nervous system, and brain in capturing reflected light from the environment and converting it to perceived images; *see also* binocular v., distance v., low v., near v., etc.

vision training: Any of several systems employing ocular exercises to enhance development or to correct deficiencies of stereopsis, hand-eye coordination, etc; *see also* orthoptics.

visual acuity (VA): Level of visual clarity; specifically, the ability to distinguish fine details, often expressed as a score on Snellen's, Jaeger's, or other vision test charts; **best corrected v.a. (BCVA)** highest level of visual acuity that can be attained with corrective lenses in place; **corrected v.a. (VA_{cc})** visual acuity measured with current corrective lenses in place; **uncorrected v.a. (UCVA or VA_{sc})** visual acuity measured without corrective lenses in place; *see also* count finger v., hand-motion v., light perception, light projection, *and* no light perception.

visual axis: Imaginary line traced from the fovea to the object of fixation, commonly called the *line of sight*.

visual evoked potential (VEP) or **visual evoked response (VER):** Fluctuation in brain activity in the visual cortex that results from a visual stimulus, measurable on electroencephalography.

visual field (VF): 1. Area around the fixation point of each eye, generally circular in shape, in which objects are perceived; 2. in clinical usage, graphs representing the result of perimetry and other such tests are often simply referred to as visual fields; visual field testing is often conducted to delineate and measure areas of the retina that are damaged (eg, by glaucoma or retinal disorders), as well as to determine any portions of the optic nerve tract that might be compromised; *see also* perimetry.

visual field defect: Area of diminished or absent vision within the visual field; **hysterical v.f.d.** apparent area of diminished or absent vision within the visual field that cannot be correlated to ocular damage or disease and, thus, seems to have an emotional basis; the isopters have a "spiral" pattern or a tube pattern that does not expand with distance from the subject; *see also* hemianopia, quadrantanopia, scotoma, *and* tunnel field.

visual pathway: Structures involved in transmitting visual stimuli, generally considered to be the optic nerve, optic chiasm, optic tract, lateral geniculate body, optic radiations, and visual cortex.

vitrectomy: Surgical procedure involving partial or total removal of vitreous humor and any membranes, blood, or other tissue in the posterior chamber; **anterior v.** vitrectomy used to remove vitreous in the anterior segment (generally present as a complication of other ocular surgery); **automated v.** vitrectomy performed using a cutting probe with irrigation and aspiration capabilities; **complete v.** removal of all vitreous from the posterior chamber; **manual v.** vitrectomy performed using scissors rather than a vitrector; **open-sky v.** vitrectomy performed by opening the cornea and removing the lens; **pars plana v.** vitrectomy performed by making small incisions and inserting instruments through the pars plana; **partial v.** removal of only part of the vitreous humor from the posterior chamber; **scissors v.** another term for manual v.; **total v.** another term for complete v.

vitrector: Surgical instrument designed for performing vitrectomy, incorporating a cutting probe with irrigation and aspiration capabilities.

vitreous body or **humor:** Clear, fibrous, gel-like material filling the posterior segment of the eye, located behind the lens capsule and comprising about two-thirds of the total volume of the eye; typically referred to simply as the *vitreous*.

vitreous detachment: Separation of all or part of the vitreous humor from its natural attachments to the retina; also called *posterior vitreous detachment (PVD)*.

vitreous face: *See* hyaloid membrane.

vitreous floaters: *See* floaters.

vitreous membrane: *See* hyaloid membrane.

vitreous strands: Vitreous humor in the anterior chamber as strands of viscous, transparent tissue still attached to the hyaloid membrane.

vitreous tap: Diagnostic procedure in which a small amount of vitreous humor is removed for testing, usually to perform a culture to confirm the existence and cause of infection.

von Graefe's sign: Delay in or absence of downward motion of upper eyelid when the eye looks downward, associated with Graves' disease (which involves serious dysfunction of the thyroid gland); *compare* pseudo-von Graefe's sign.

vortex veins: Veins formed by the joining of veins draining blood from the iris, ciliary body, and choroid exiting the eye through the sclera just posterior to the equator of the globe.

W

wall-eye: Common term for exotropia.

Weck-cel sponge: Brand name (Pilling Weck, Fort Washington, Pa) of a widely used surgical instrument consisting of a wedge of cellulose sponge mounted on a short handle; some procedures, most notably Weck-cel vitrectomy, in which the sponge plays a major role, are identified using the term.

wet macular degeneration: *See* macular degeneration.

wetting angle: Angle between the surface of a drop of water and the surface of the material on which the drop lies; in ophthalmic usage, usually a description of contact lens materials, referring to the spread of moisture on the lens surface; the smaller the contact angle, the more hydrophilic or "wettable" the material.

white-to-white measurement: Diameter of the cornea as measured from the edges of white scleral tissue.

with-the-rule (WTR) astigmatism: *See* astigmatism.

working lens: Plus-powered lens used during retinoscopy to compensate for the distance between examiner and patient; with a working distance of 66 cm, the power of the working lens is +1.50 diopters; the power of the working lens must be subtracted from the final reading in order to obtain the patient's refractive error.

Worth 4-dot or **Worth four-dot test (W4D):** Test of binocular vision or suppression; four illuminated dots (colored white, red, and green) are presented to the patient, who views them through glasses with one red and one green lens.

xanthelasma/xanthoma: Yellowish, raised, benign growth composed of fatty tissue, generally found on the upper lids but sometimes on the lower; may be associated with elevated cholesterol.

xenon photocoagulator: Device that produces intensely bright light, with ophthalmic applications similar to lasers.

xenophthalmia: General term for unhealthy condition of an eye attributable to the presence of a foreign body.

xerophthalmia: Dry eye condition in which the conjunctiva thickens and atrophies and the eye lacks luster.

xerosis: General term referring to tissue dryness.

Y-sutures (of crystalline lens): Tissue structure of the crystalline lens in which the ends of nuclear and cortical fibers join to form a Y shape; the anterior Y is upright and the posterior is inverted.

YAG laser: *See* Nd:YAG laser *under* laser.

yoke muscles: Two extraocular muscles (one of each eye) that are neurologically paired so that they coordinate motion of both eyes in the same direction; also called *synergists*; *see also* Hering's law of simultaneous innervation.

Z

Zeis' glands: Oil-producing glands within the eyelids that empty into eyelash follicles.

Zeiss lens: *See* goniolens.

zonules: Fibers that attach the edge of the lens capsule to the ciliary body.

zonulolysis or **zonulysis:** Breakage of the zonules, occurring either naturally (from trauma) or through intentional or unintentional surgical manipulation.

zygomatic bone: One of the bones of the orbit.

LIST OF APPENDICES

Appendix 1:   Acronyms and Abbreviations. . . . 195
Appendix 2:   Medical Terminology 209
Appendix 3:   The Schematic Eye. 215
Appendix 4:   The Cranial Nerves 217
Appendix 5:   Classifications of Nystagmus 219
Appendix 6:   Red Eye Differential Diagnosis . . 221
Appendix 7:   The Subjective Grading System . . 225
Appendix 8:   Slit Lamp Findings for Systemic
                Diseases and Conditions. 233
Appendix 9:   Systemic Disorders and Their
                Effects On the Eye 239
Appendix 10:   Ophthalmic Drugs. 247
Appendix 11:   Lasers in Ophthalmology 279
Appendix 12:   Ocular and Systemic Effects
                of Topical Ocular Drugs 283
Appendix 13:   Normal Values of Common
                Blood Tests. 287
Appendix 14:   The Metric System. 289
Appendix 15:   English and Metric Conversion . . 293
Appendix 16:   Weights and Measures 295
Appendix 17:   Manual Alphabet for
                Communicating With the
                Hearing Impaired 297
Appendix 18:   The Braille Alphabet 299
Appendix 19:   Certification as Paraoptometric
                and Ophthalmic Medical
                Personnel 301
Appendix 20:   Websites Related to Eyecare 309
Appendix 21:   Suggested Reading 321

ACRONYMS AND ABBREVIATIONS

2°IOL: secondary IOL
2°OAG: secondary open-angle glaucoma
5-FU: 5-fluorouracil
Δ: prism, change

A: applanation tonometry (also AT)
AA: accommodative amplitude
AAO: American Academy of Ophthalmology, American Academy of Optometry
ABES: American Board of Eye Surgeons
ABK: aphakic bullous keratopathy
ABO: American Board of Ophthalmology, American Board of Opticianry
ac: before meals
AC: anterior chamber, accommodative convergence
AC/A: accommodative convergence/accommodation (ratio)
ACES: American College of Eye Surgeons
ACG: angle-closure glaucoma
A/CIOL: anterior chamber intraocular lens implant
ACL: anterior chamber (intraocular) lens (implant)
ACS: American College of Surgeons, Automated Corneal Shaper (trademarked microkeratome)
AG: Amsler grid
AI: accommodative insufficiency
AIDS: acquired immunodeficiency syndrome
AK: astigmatic keratotomy, actinic keratosis, arcuate keratotomy, automated lamellar keratoplasty
ALK: automated lamellar keratoplasty
ALT: argon laser trabeculoplasty
AMA: American Medical Association

AMD: age-related macular degeneration
AMO: Allergan Medical Optics (company name)
ANSI: American National Standards Institute
AOA: American Optometric Association
AOZ: anterior optical zone
AOZD: anterior optic zone diameter
Ap: applanation tonometry
APD: afferent pupillary defect (Marcus Gunn pupil)
AR: autorefraction
ARC: abnormal or anomalous retinal correspondence
ARE: acute red eye
ARMD: age-related macular degeneration
ARP: Argyll Robertson pupil
asb: apostilb
ASC: anterior subcapsular cataract
ASCRS: American Society of Cataract and Refractive Surgery
ASICO: American Surgical Instrument Company
astig: astigmatism
AT: applanation tonometry, artificial tears
ATPO: Association of Technical Personnel in Ophthalmology
ATR: against-the-rule (astigmatism)
AUPO: Association of University Professors in Ophthalmology

B9: benign
BAK: benzalkonium chloride
BAT: Brightness Acuity Tester (trademark)
BC: base curve
BCC: basal cell carcinoma
BCVA: best corrected visual acuity
BD: base down (prism)
BDR: background diabetic retinopathy
BI: base in (prism)
bid: twice daily
BIOM: Binocular Indirect Ophthalmic Microscope (trademark)

BLL: brow, lids, lashes
BM: basement membrane
BO: base out (prism)
BRA: branch retinal artery
BRAO: branch retinal artery occlusion
BRB: blood-retinal barrier
BRV: branch retinal vein
BRVO: branch retinal vein occlusion
BSD: back surface debris
BSS: balanced salt solution
BTX: Botulinum toxin
BU: base up (prism)
BUT: break-up time (tear test)
BUVA: best uncorrected visual acuity
BVP: back vertex power

C_3F_8: perfluoropropane
c: with
C/F: cell/flare
CA: carcinoma
CAC: central anterior curve
CACT: computer-assisted corneal topography
CAI: carbonic anhydrase inhibitor
caps: capsule
CAT: computerized tomography (CT scan)
cd: candela
c/d: cup-to-disc ratio
CE: cataract extraction, complete exam
CE/IOL: cataract extraction with intraocular lens implant
CF: count fingers, cystic fibrosis
CI: convergence insufficiency
CL: contact lens
CLAO: Contact Lens Association of Ophthalmologists
clr: clear
cm: centimeter
CME: cystoid macular edema
CMV: cytomegalovirus

CN: cranial nerve
CN II: second cranial nerve (optic nerve)
CN III: third cranial nerve (oculomotor nerve)
CN IV: fourth cranial nerve (trochlear nerve)
CN V: fifth cranial nerve (trigeminal nerve)
CN VI: sixth cranial nerve (abducens nerve)
CN VII: seventh cranial nerve (facial nerve)
CNS: central nervous system
CNV: choroidal neovascularization
CO: certified orthoptist, corneal opacity
CO$_2$: carbon dioxide
COA: certified ophthalmic assistant
COAG: chronic open-angle glaucoma
coll/collyr: eyewash
COMT: certified ophthalmic medical technologist
conj: conjunctiva, conjunctivitis
COT: certified ophthalmic technician
CPC: central posterior curve
CPOA: certified paraoptometric assistant
CPOT: certified paraoptometric technician
CRA: central retinal artery
CRAO: central retinal artery occlusion
CRNO: certified registered nurse in ophthalmology
CRP: corneal reflection pupillometer
CRV: central retinal vein
CRVO: central retinal vein occlusion
CSR: central serous retinopathy
CST: contrast sensitivity test
CT: center thickness (contact lens), computed tomography (CAT scan)
CTL: contact lens(es)
CWS: cotton-wool spot
cyl: cylinder

d: day
D: disc, diopter(s), distance, diameter
D&C: deep and clear

D&Q: deep and quiet
D/N: distance and at near
dB: decibel
DBC: distance between centers
DBL: distance between lenses
DC: dermatochalasis, discharge, discontinue, diopters (of) cylinder
DCR: dacryocystorhinostomy
dd: disc diameter
Deq: spherical equivalent
DES: dry eye syndrome, disc edges sharp
Dk: oxygen permeability
Dk/L: oxygen transmissibility
DM: diabetes mellitus
DR: diabetic retinopathy
DS: diopter(s) sphere
DVD: dissociated vertical deviation

E: esophoria, eccentricity
E': esophoria at near
ECCE: extracapsular cataract extraction
ED: epithelial defect, effective diameter
EDTA: ethylenediaminetetraacetate
EEG: electroencephalography
EKC: epidemic keratoconjunctivitis
EOG: electro-oculogram
EOM: extraocular muscle(s)
Er:YAG: erbium:yttrium-aluminum-garnet (laser)
ERG: electroretinogram
ERM: epiretinal membrane
ET: esotropia, edge thickness (contact lenses)
ET': esotropia at near
E(T): intermittent esotropia
EUA: exam under anesthesia
Excimer: excited dimer laser

F&F: fix and follow

FA: fluorescein angiogram

FAAO: Fellow of the American Academy of Ophthalmology, Fellow of the American Academy of Optometry

FACS: Fellow of the American College of Surgeons

FAP: flatter add plus

FAZ: foveal avascular zone

FB: foreign body

FDA: Food and Drug Administration

FRCP: Fellow of the Royal College of Physicians (of England)

FRCPA: Fellow of the Royal College of Physicians (of Australia)

FRCPC: Fellow of the Royal College of Physicians (of Canada)

FRCS: Fellow of the Royal College of Surgeons (of England)

FRCSA: Fellow of the Royal College of Surgeons (of Australia)

FRCSC: Fellow of the Royal College of Surgeons (of Canada)

FTC: full to confrontation

GCD: geometric center distance

GCM: good, central, maintained

GCNM: good, central, not maintained

GFE: gas-fluid exchange

GPC: giant papillary conjunctivitis

GPCL: gas-permeable contact lens

gt: drop

gtt: drops

h: hour

HE: hard exudate

HEMA: hydroxyethylmethacrylate

HeNe: helium-neon (laser)

Hg: mercury
HIV: human immunodeficiency virus
HM: hand motion
HOTV: H, O, T, and V letter test
HRC: high risk characteristics, harmonious retinal correspondence
hs: at bedtime
HSK: herpes simplex keratitis
HSV: herpes simplex virus
HVF: Humphrey visual field (Humphrey Instruments, San Leandro, Calif)

i: one
ii: two
iii: three
I&R: insertion and removal (contact lens)
IA, I/A, I&A: irrigation and aspiration
ICCE: intracapsular cataract extraction
ICE: iridocorneal endothelial syndrome
ICG: indocyanine green
ICL: Implantable Contact Lens (tradename)
ICR: Intrastromal Corneal Ring (tradename), intermediate curve (contact lens)
IDDM: insulin-dependent diabetes mellitus
Ig: immunoglobulin
IK: interstitial keratitis
ILM: internal limiting membrane
IO: inferior oblique
IOFB: intraocular foreign body
IOL: intraocular lens (implant)
ION: ischemic optic neuropathy
IOP: intraocular pressure
IPD: interpupillary distance
IR: inferior rectus, index of refraction
ISRS: International Society of Refractive Surgery

J: Jaeger
JCAHPO: Joint Commission on Allied Health Personnel in Ophthalmology
JND: just noticeable difference
JRA: juvenile rheumatoid arthritis

K: cornea, keratometry, keratometric value
KC: keratoconus
KCS: keratoconjunctivitis sicca
KP: keratitic precipitate
KPE: Kelman phacoemulsification

L: center thickness (contact lens)
LARS: left add/right subtract
LARP: laser reversal of presbyopia (also LRP)
Laser: light amplification by stimulated emission of radiation
LASIK: laser-assisted in-situ keratomileusis
LE: left eye
LEC: lens epithelial cells
LGV: lymphogranuloma venereum
LHT: left hypertropia
LIO: left inferior oblique, laser indirect ophthalmoscope
LK: lamellar keratoplasty
LKP: lamellar keratoplasty (also LK)
LLL: left lower lid
LP: light perception
LP w/proj: LP with projection
LP w/o proj: LP without projection
LR: lateral rectus
LRP: laser reversal of myopia (also LARP)
LTG: low tension glaucoma
LTK: laser thermal keratoplasty
LUL: left upper lid
LV: low vision
LVS: low vision specialist
LXT: left exotropia

m: meter
MA: macroaneurysm, manifest astigmatism
MD: macular degeneration, medical doctor
MDF: Map-Dot-Fingerprint dystrophy
ME: macular edema
MG: Marcus Gunn pupil, myasthenia gravis
mm: millimeter
mmHg: millimeters of mercury
Motcc: motility with correction
Motsc: motility without correction
MR: manifest refraction, medial rectus
MRI: magnetic resonance imaging
MS: multiple sclerosis
MTF: modulation transfer function
MVL: moderate visual loss

N: near
NaFl: sodium fluorescein
NAG: narrow-angle glaucoma
NCLE: National Contact Lens Examiners
NCT: noncontact tonometry
Nd:YAG: neodymium:yttrium-aluminum-garnet (laser)
NEI: National Eye Institute
neo: neovascularization
NFL: nerve fiber layer
NIDDM: noninsulin-dependent diabetes mellitus
NIH: National Institutes of Health
NLD: nasolacrimal duct
NLP: no light perception
nm: nanometer
NPA: near point of accommodation
NPC: near point of convergence
NPDR: nonproliferative diabetic retinopathy
npo: nothing by mouth
NRC: normal retinal correspondence
NS: nuclear sclerosis
NSAID: nonsteroidal anti-inflammatory drug

NSPB: National Society for the Prevention of Blindness
NTG: normal tension glaucoma
NVA: near visual acuity
NVG: neovascular glaucoma

OA: overaction (as in muscles), ophthalmic artery, optometric assistant, ophthalmic assistant
OAG: open-angle glaucoma
OC: optical center
OCT: Optical Coherence Tomographer (trademark)
OD: oculus dexter (right eye), doctor of optometry
ODM: ophthalmodynamometry
OEP: Optometric Extension Program
OHS: ocular histoplasmosis syndrome
OHT: ocular hypertension
OKN: optokinetic nystagmus
ON: optic nerve, optic neuritis, optic neuropathy
OOSS: Outpatient Ophthalmic Surgery Society
Ortho-K: orthokeratology
OS: oculus sinister (left eye)
OSHA: Occupational Safety and Health Administration
OT: ophthalmic technician, optometric technician
OU: oculus uterque (both eyes together)
OZ: optical zone
OZD: optic zone diameter
OZR: optic zone radius

P: periphery, pupils
P&I: probe and irrigate
PAL: progressive addition lens
PAM: Potential Acuity Meter (trademark)
PARK: photorefractive astigmatic keratectomy
PAS: peripheral anterior synechia
PBK: pseudophakic bullous keratopathy
pc: after meals
PC: posterior capsule, posterior chamber
PCIOL: posterior chamber intraocular lens (implant)

PCL: posterior chamber (intraocular) lens (implant)
PCO: posterior capsule opacification
PCR: posterior curve
PD: prism diopters, pupillary distance
PDR: proliferative diabetic retinopathy
PDT: photodynamic therapy
PEE: punctate epithelial erosions
PERRLA: pupils equally round and reactive to light and accommodation
pH: refers to the acidic or basic property of a substance
PH: pinhole
phaco: phacoemulsification
PI: peripheral iridotomy, peripheral iridectomy
PK: penetrating keratoplasty
PKP: penetrating keratoplasty
pl: plano
PMMA: polymethylmethacrylate
po: by mouth
POAG: primary open-angle glaucoma
POZD: posterior optic zone diameter
PRK: photorefractive keratectomy
prn: as needed
PRP: panretinal photocoagulation
PS: posterior synechia
PSC: posterior subcapsular cataract
PTK: phototherapeutic keratectomy
PVD: posterior vitreous detachment
PVR: proliferative vitreoretinopathy

q: every
q2h: every 2 hours
qd: every day
qh: every hour
qid: four times a day
qs: as much as needed

R&R: recess and resect
RA: rheumatoid arthritis
RAPD: relative afferent pupillary defect
RD: retinal detachment
RE: right eye
RGP: rigid gas permeable (contact lens)
RHT: right hypertropia
RK: radial keratotomy
RLF: retrolental fibroplasia (now ROP)
RLL: right lower lid
ROP: retinopathy of prematurity (was RLF)
RP: retinitis pigmentosa
RPE: retinal pigment epithelium
rpm: revolutions per minute
RUL: right upper lid
Rx: prescribe

s or sine: without
SAM: steeper add minus
SB: scleral buckle
SCH: subconjunctival hemorrhage
SCL: soft contact lens
SCO: spherocylindrical over-refraction
SCR: secondary curve
SE: soft exudates, side effects, spherical equivalent
SEI: subepithelial infiltrates
SF_6: sulfur hexafluoride
sig: instructions
SLE: slit lamp exam, systemic lupus erythematosus
SLK: superior limbic keratoconjunctivitis
SMD: senile macular degeneration
SO: superior oblique, sympathetic ophthalmia
sol: solution
sph: spherical correction
SPK: superficial punctate keratitis
SR: superior rectus
SRP: surgical reversal of presbyopia

ST: straight top (bifocal/trifocal)
susp: suspension
SVL: severe visual loss
SVP: spontaneous venous pulsations

T: tonometry, tropia
tab: tablet
TB: tuberculosis
tid: three times daily
TK: thermokeratoplasty
TM: trabecular meshwork
Tp: Tono-Pen (trademark)
TRIC: trachoma inclusion conjunctivitis

UA: underaction (as in muscles)
UCVA: uncorrected visual acuity (also VA_{sc})
UGH: uveitis, glaucoma, hyphema syndrome
ung: ointment
ut dict: as directed
UV: ultraviolet light
UVA: ultraviolet band A
UVB: ultraviolet band B

V: visual acuity, versions
VA: visual acuity
VA_{cc}: visual acuity with correction
VA_{sc}: visual acuity without correction
VEP: visual evoked potential
VER: visual evoked response
VF: visual field(s)
VH: vitreous hemorrhage

w/u: work-up
W4D: Worth 4-Dot test
WHO: World Health Organization
WNL: within normal limits
WTR: with-the-rule (astigmatism)

X: exophoria
X′: exophoria at near
X(T): intermittent exotropia
XT: exotropia
XT′: exotropia at near

YAG: yttrium-aluminum-garnet (laser)

Medical Terminology

The good news about medical terminology is that you do not have to memorize hundreds of words. Medical terms are put together using a system... so if you know the system, you do not have to memorize a lot of words. The basis for most of these terms is Greek or Latin, but a good number of them are already in your everyday vocabulary. Many medical and anatomical terms are made up of words put together. It is just like putting English words together.

All words are built around a root word, with the root word acting as the foundation (eg, ogle, yawn, destiny). Some words are made up of two root words; these are called *compound words* (eg, sometimes, applesauce, joystick).

We also use prefixes (ie, the word part that comes *before* a word [eg, pre-, un-]) and suffixes (ie, the word part that comes *after* a word [eg, -er, -ed, -ing]) with root words both in daily conversation and medical terminology.

A root word may be joined with a combining form to make a compound word. In medical terminology, the combining form is usually a vowel. You already know how to do this, whether you realize it or not. Take the word thermometer. *Therm/o*, using the combining form (o), refers to the temperature. The suffix *–meter* means a device used to measure.

Medical words are generally built from a root word, a combining form, and an ending of some sort. If you know the meaning of the root word and the prefix or suffix, you can pretty much figure out any medical or scientific term.

Compound words using combining forms are *built*. Suppose you needed a word that meant skimming over the surface of the water. *Hydr/o* for water, *-plane* for surface = hydroplane. What if you were afraid of water? *Hydrophobia*. Suppose you saw the word *photophobia* and didn't know what it meant. You see *–phobia* and you know that it means an unnatural fear of something. What does *phot/o* make you think of? Maybe photograph, but this is not a fear of photographs… it's a fear of light. Now that you know that *phot/o* means light, you could figure out *photopsia*. It has something to do with light… *-opsia* refers to vision. So literally, it is a vision of light. Fancy name for light flashes and other such sparkles!

Let's play with this a minute. The suffix *–itis* means inflammation. *Tonsillitis, gingivitis, cystitis*. How many eye-related inflammatory words can you think of? *Blepharitis, conjunctivitis, scleritis, episcleritis, uveitis,* and *iritis* are just a few. They are inflammations of the lids, conjunctiva, sclera, episclera, uvea, and iris, respectively.

Below are some combining forms, prefixes, and suffixes useful in eye care.

ROOT WORDS RELATED TO OCULAR ANATOMY

blephar/o	lids
bulb/a	globe; eyeball
cili/o	eyelash
corne/o	cornea
cycl/o	ciliary body
dacry/o	tear
dermat/o	skin
ir/i	iris
kerat/o	cornea
lacrim/a	tear
ophthalm/o	eye
phak/o	lens
retin/o	retina

scler/o	sclera
tars/o	tarsal plate
trich	hair
uve-	uvea

Root Words Related to Vision, Eyes, Etc

ambl/y	dim, dull
astigmat	without a point
dipl/o	double
hyper/o	above, over, excessive
-ism	condition with a specific cause
my/o	to shut
ocul/o	eye
-opia	vision
-opsia	vision
opsis	vision
opt/o, optic/o	vision
phot/o	light
presby/o	old man

Root Words Related to Surgery

cente-	puncture
-cis-	cut
cry/o	cold
-ectomy	excise or remove a part
-orrhaphy	suturing or stitching
-ostomy	form an opening
-otomy	incise or cut into a part
-plasty	surgical repair of

Other Useful
Root Words, Prefixes, and Suffixes

a-, an-	without
ab-	away from

ad-	toward
angi/o	blood vessel
anis/o	without equality, unequal
anti-	against
aut/o	self
carcin/o	cancer
cyst/o	bladder; any sac containing fluid
-duct	lead, conduct
dys-	bad, improper, malfunction, difficult
e-	out from
-emia	blood
end/o	within
epi-	upon, after, in addition
es/o	inside
ex/o	out, outside
extra-	outside of, beyond
gram/o	record, write
graph/o	instrument used to make a record
-graphy	actual making of a record
hem/o	blood
hemat/o	blood
hemi	half
heter/o	different
hom/o	same, common
hydr/o	pertaining to water
hyper-	over, above, beyond
hypo-	under, below
-iasis	condition, pathological state
-ism	condition, theory
is/o	equal
-itis	inflammation
-lysis	disintegration
macr/o	larger than normal
mal-	bad, abnormal

megal/o	great, large
-meter	measure
micr/o	smaller than normal
mon/o	only, sole, single
morph	shape, form
mot-	move
mult/i	many
my/o	muscle
nas/o	nose
ne/o	new, young
neur/o	nerves
-oma	tumor
orth/o	straight
-osis	condition, disease
path/o, -pathy	disease
phob/o, -phobia	abnormal fear of
phor-	motion, carrying
-plegia	paralysis
pseud/o	false
ptosis	prolapse
punct-	pierce, prick
quadr-	four
schis-	split
-spasm	twitch
-scope	instrument for examining
-scopy	examining with a scope
spectr-	appearance, what is seen
sym-, syn-	with, together
therm-	heat
ton/o-	tone, pressure
tors-	twist
trop-	turn
uni-	one
vers-	turn
vert-	turn

ROOT WORDS AND PREFIXES
RELATED TO COLORS

alb-	white
chrom/o	color
cyan/o	blue
erythr/o	red
leuk/o	white
melan/o	black
xanth/o	yellow

PREFIXES RELATED TO LOCATION, TIME, ETC

ab-	away from
endo-	within, inner
infra-	below
pan-	entire, all
peri-	around
post-	after
pre-	before
retro-	behind
sub-	under, below
supra-	above

The Schematic Eye

STRUCTURE	NOTES
Cornea	IR = 1.376
	Radius of central anterior surface = 7.7 mm
	Radius of posterior surface = 6.8 mm
	Refractive power of anterior surface = +48.83 D
	Refractive power of posterior surface = -5.88 D
	Total refractive power = +42.95 D
	Central thickness = 0.5 mm
Pupil	"Ideal" size = 2 to 5 mm
Aqueous	IR = 1.336
Lens	IR of cortex = 1.386
	IR of nucleus = 1.406
	Overall IR = 1.42
	Anterior radius of curvature (unaccommodated) = 10.00 mm
	Anterior radius of curvature (fully accommodated) = 5.33 mm
	Posterior radius of curvature (unaccommodated) = 6.0 mm
	Posterior radius of curvature (fully accommodated) = 5.3 mm
	Refractive power (unaccommodated) = +19 D
	Refractive power (fully accommodated) = +33.06 D

STRUCTURE	NOTES
	Thickness of nucleus = 2.419 mm
	Overall thickness = 3.6 mm
Vitreous	IR = 1.336
Axial length	Overall eye length = 24.4 mm
	Distance from anterior K to anterior lens surface = 3.6 mm
	Distance from anterior K to posterior lens surface = 7.2 mm
	Distance from posterior lens surface to retina = 17.2 mm

IR = index of refraction; D = diopters; K = cornea

Reprinted with permission from Ledford J. *Certified Ophthalmic Medical Technologist Exam Review Manual.* Thorofare, NJ: SLACK Incorporated; 1997: 153.

The Cranial Nerves

CRANIAL NERVE	NAME	MOTOR/FUNCTION	SENSORY
I	Olfactory	Sensory	Smell
II	Optic	Sensory	Sight
III	Oculomotor	Motor	Movement of eye (MR, SR, IR, and IO), pupil constriction, accommodation, and upper lid elevation
IV	Trochlear	Motor	Superior oblique muscle
V	Trigeminal	Mixed	Sensation of touch in face, nose, forehead, temple, tongue, and eye; innervation for chewing
VI	Abducens	Motor	Lateral rectus muscle

CRANIAL NERVE	NAME	MOTOR/ FUNCTION	SENSORY
VII	Facial	Mixed	Reflex tearing, facial expression, some taste, and blinking
VIII	Vestibulocochlear (acoustic nerve)	Sensory	Hearing and equilibrium
IX	Glossopharyngeal	Mixed	Taste and swallowing
X	Vagus	Mixed	Taste, heart rate, breathing, digestion, and voice
XI	Spinal accessory	Motor	Innervation of neck and shoulder muscles, provides posture and rotation of head
XII	Hypoglossal	Motor	Tongue movement

MR = medial rectus muscle; SR = superior rectus muscle; IR = inferior rectus muscle; and IO = inferior oblique muscle

Reprinted with permission from Lens A, Langley T, Nemeth SC, Shea C. *Ocular Anatomy and Physiology*. Thorofare, NJ: SLACK Incorporated; 1999.

Classifications of Nystagmus

I. Normal physiologic
   A. Endpoint
   B. Induced
      1. Drugs
      2. Optokinetic
      3. Caloric
      4. Rotational
II. Congenital
   A. Motor (idiopathic)
   B. Sensory (sensory vision)
   C. Latent
III. Acquired
   A. Convergence retraction
   B. Cerebellar
      1. Opsoclonus
      2. Flutter
      3. Dysmetria
   C. Gaze—paretic
   D. Vestibular
      1. Rotary
      2. Horizontal
      3. Vertical
   E. Spasmus nutans
   F. Muscle—paretic
   G. See-saw
   H. Periodic alternating

Adapted from Cassin B, ed. *Fundamentals for Ophthalmic Technical Personnel.* Philadelphia, Pa: WB Saunders; 1995.

Red Eye Differential Diagnosis

	CONJUNCTIVITIS	IRITIS	ACUTE ANGLE-CLOSURE GLAUCOMA	KERATITIS, CORNEAL FOREIGN BODY
Vision	Normal to blurring that clears with blinking	Mild blurring	Considerable blurring or haziness; halos around lights	Mild blurring
Pain	None to minor discomfort, burning, or grittiness	Moderate to aching	Severe aching	Sharp pain or foreign body sensation
Discharge	Dependent on type: Mucopurulent—bacterial Watery—viral Watery/stringy—allergic	None	None	None to mild

	CONJUNCTIVITIS	IRITIS	ACUTE ANGLE-CLOSURE GLAUCOMA	KERATITIS, CORNEAL FOREIGN BODY
Pattern of redness	Palpebral conjunctival and/or diffuse conjunctival	Conjunctival circumcorneal pattern	Diffuse conjunctival with prominent circumcorneal pattern	Conjunctival circumcorneal pattern
Pupil (affected eye)	Normal, reactive	Constricted—may be slightly reactive	Dilated, fixed	Normal to constricted, reactive
Cornea	Clear	Clear to slightly hazy	Hazy	Possible visible FB opacification, abnormal light reflex, fluorescein staining
IOP	Normal	Normal to low	High	Normal

	CONJUNCTIVITIS	IRITIS	ACUTE ANGLE-CLOSURE GLAUCOMA	KERATITIS, CORNEAL FOREIGN BODY
Other		Photophobia	Possible nausea and vomiting	Possible photophobia

Reprinted with permission from Hargis-Greenshields L, Sims L. *Emergencies in Eyecare*. Thorofare, NJ: SLACK Incorporated; 1999.

The Subjective Grading System

An important, but confusing, part of documenting abnormalities is the subjective grading system. Even the term *subjective* causes confusion because such grading occurs during the objective examination. Some clarification seems to be in order.

First, many of the patient's symptoms are subjective. These are symptoms that the patient tells us about but we cannot see, such as pain. Other findings are objective. That is, they do not involve the patient's ability to report them. We can see them ourselves when we examine the patient. Cell and flare in the anterior chamber is an objective finding; the patient did not (and cannot) tell us about it, but we can see it. Other findings fall into both realms. The patient may say, "My right eye is red," which is subjective. We can also see the injection through the slit lamp (whether the patient has reported it or not), which is objective. The slit lamp exam is an objective test.

Grading pathology and other findings, although they are discovered during the *objective* examination, are *subjective* on the part of the examiner. By subjective we mean that the assignment of a rating to a finding is dependent on the observer's opinion. You may look at the patient and grade her lid edema as 2+. Another clinician may rate the same finding (same patient, same day, and same time) as 1+ or 3+. The best we can advise you is that if you are auxiliary personnel, try to learn the grading system of your employer. As you examine more and more eyes, you will get a feel for how marked a finding is. If you are a physician, do your best to teach your grading philosophy to your staff.

With that said, we would like to offer our own opinion about how to grade your findings. Some prefer a numbered grading system. If you use this, then 0+ means that a finding is absent. 1+ would indicate that a finding is just barely perceptible. 4+ would refer to a full-blown case. Using this schematic, 2+ and 3+ would fall somewhere in between. Interjecting half steps in between, such as 2.5+, sometimes complicates this system. We will leave it up to you as to whether this practice is truly necessary or not.

Instead of numbers, specific terms can be used, including "none, absent, bare trace, trace, slight, moderate, marked, severe," and other such words. This is even more subjective than the numbering system. If everyone uses a scale of 0 to 4, then we have a better chance of understanding what 2+ means. Who is to say what the difference really is between "bare trace" and "trace"? (Alas, perhaps it is that nebulous 0.5 half-step!) The dilemma of subjective grading is not likely to be resolved.

GRADING INJECTION

Features	*Grade*
No injection present	0
Slight limbal (mild segmented), bulbar (mild regional), and/or palpebral injection	1
Mild limbal (mild circumcorneal), bulbar (mild diffuse), and/or palpebral injection	2
Significant limbal (marked segmented), bulbar (marked regional or diffuse), or palpebral injection	3
Severe limbal (marked circumcorneal), bulbar (diffuse episcleral or scleral), or palpebral injection	4

Adapted from FDA document *Premarket Notification Guidance Document for Daily Wear Contact Lenses*. Reprinted with permission from Ledford JK, Sanders VN. *The Slit Lamp Primer*. Thorofare, NJ: SLACK Incorporated; 1998.

GRADING CORNEAL HAZE

Features	*Grade*
Clear	0
Between clear and trace; barely perceptible	0.5+
Trace; easily seen with slit lamp	1+
Mild haze	2+

Features	Grade
Moderate haze, very pronounced, iris details still visible, anterior chamber (AC) reaction not visible	3+
Marked haze, scarring, iris details obscured	4+

Adapted from Stein HA, Cheskes AT, Stein RM. *The Excimer: Fundamentals & Clinical Use.* Thorofare, NJ: SLACK Incorporated; 1995.

GRADING CORNEAL VASCULARIZATION

Features	Grade
No vascular changes	0
Congestion and dilation of the limbal vessels; single vessel extension < 1.5 mm	1
Extension of multiple vessels < 1.5 mm	2
Extension of multiple limbal vessels 1.5 to 2.5 mm	3
Segmented or circumscribed extension of limbal vessels > 2.5 mm or to within 3.0 mm of corneal apex	4

Adapted from FDA document *Premarket Notification Guidance Document for Daily Wear Contact Lenses.* Reprinted with permission from Ledford JK, Sanders VN. *The Slit Lamp Primer.* Thorofare, NJ: SLACK Incorporated; 1998.

The Subjective Grading System

GRADING CORNEAL STAINING

Features	Grade
No staining	0
Minimal superficial staining or stippling	1
Regional or diffuse punctate staining	2
Significant dense coalesced staining, corneal abrasion, or foreign body tracks	3
Severe abrasions > 2 mm diameter, ulcerations, epithelial loss, or full-thickness abrasion	4

Adapted from FDA document *Premarket Notification Guidance Document for Daily Wear Contact Lenses*. Reprinted with permission from Ledford JK, Sanders VN. *The Slit Lamp Primer*. Thorofare, NJ: SLACK Incorporated; 1998.

GRADING ANGLES

Features	Grade
Closed angle	0
Angle extremely narrow, probable closure	1+
Angle moderately narrow, possible closure	2+
Angle moderately open, closure not possible	3+
Angle wide open, closure not possible	4+

Reprinted with permission from Ledford JK, Sanders VN. *The Slit Lamp Primer*. Thorofare, NJ: SLACK Incorporated; 1998.

GRADING CELL (1 MM CONICAL BEAM)

Cell #	Grade
1 to 10	Trace
10 to 20	1+
20 to 30	2+
30 to 40	3+
40 up to hypopyon	4+

Reprinted with permission from Ledford JK, Sanders VN. *The Slit Lamp Primer.* Thorofare, NJ: SLACK Incorporated; 1998.

GRADING CORTICAL CATARACTS

Features	Grade
Gray lines, dots, and flakes aligned along the cortical fibers in periphery; visible in oblique direct illumination	1+ (early or incipient)
Opaque spokes, anterior chamber may be shallower than normal for patient	2+ (immature or intumescent)
Cortex opaque up to capsule, anterior chamber may be normal depth	3+ (mature)
Lens is smaller, wrinkly capsule, nucleus may float in liquified cortex	4+ (hyperma-ture)

Reprinted with permission from Ledford JK, Sanders VN. *The Slit Lamp Primer.* Thorofare, NJ: SLACK Incorporated; 1998.

GRADING NUCLEAR SCLEROTIC CATARACTS

Lens Color	Grade
Gray-blue (normal)	0
Yellow overtone	1+
Light amber	2+
Reddish brown	3+
Brown or black, opaque; no fundus reflection	4+

Reprinted with permission from Ledford JK, Sanders VN. *The Slit Lamp Primer.* Thorofare, NJ: SLACK Incorporated; 1998.

GRADING POSTERIOR SUBCAPSULAR CATARACTS

Features	Grade
Optical irregularity on posterior capsule; visible only on retroillumination	1+
Small, white fleck	2+ (early)
Enlarged plaque; round or irregular borders	3+ (moderate)
Opaque plaque	4+ (advanced)

Reprinted with permission from Ledford JK, Sanders VN. *The Slit Lamp Primer.* Thorofare, NJ: SLACK Incorporated; 1998.

Slit Lamp Findings for Systemic Diseases and Conditions

Some of these findings are admittedly rare.

Conjunctivitis *can include conjunctival redness, conjunctival edema, excessive tearing, and matter/discharge.*

See also notes on medications used to treat these conditions (Appendix 12).

For other complications of systemic disorders, see *Appendix 9.*

abuse (physical): Lid bruises and swelling, lid burns, subconjunctival hemorrhage (may be numerous and tiny), corneal abrasion, hyphema, traumatic cataract, lens subluxation.

acne: *See* rosacea.

acquired immunodeficiency syndrome (AIDS): Exophthalmos; conjunctivitis (recurrent infections); dry eye; Kaposi's sarcoma (reddish-blue vascular nodules) of lids, palpebral conjunctiva, or orbit.

albinism: Nystagmus, white brows and lashes, reddish iris.

alcoholism: Ptosis, nystagmus, iris paralysis.

allergies: Conjunctivitis, congestion of conjunctival blood vessels, dry eye (secondary to medication), iritis (seasonal).

anemia: Subconjunctival hemorrhage.

ankylosing spondylitis: Iritis.

arteriosclerosis: Arcus senilis.

asthma: Conjunctivitis, cataract (secondary to corticosteroid treatment).

Bell's palsy: Incomplete or absent lid closure, exposure keratitis.

breast cancer: Metastatic lesion to angle, metastatic lesion to iris, other metastatic lesions (visible mass, redness), symptoms of metastatic lesions (exophthalmos, hyphema).

cancer: *See* breast cancer, colon cancer, leukemia, lung cancer, and melanoma.

Candida albicans (yeast): Swelling of lacrimal gland, lid "thrush," conjunctivitis, stringy mucus, keratitis, pseudomembranes.

carotid artery disease: Dilation of conjunctival blood vessels, iritis.

chickenpox: Vesicles on lid, conjunctivitis, abnormal pupil, superficial punctate keratitis, iritis.

Chlamydia: Lid swelling, conjunctival injection, conjunctivitis, conjunctival pseudomembranes, keratitis, corneal vascularization.

colon cancer: Metastatic lesions (visible mass, redness), symptoms of metastatic lesions (exophthalmos, hyphema).

craniofacial syndromes: Exophthalmos, nystagmus, exposure keratitis, coloboma.

diabetes: Xanthelasma, corneal wrinkles, rubeosis of iris, loss of iris pigment, cataract, asteroid hyalosis.

Down syndrome: Nystagmus, epicanthal folds, keratoconus, iris spots, Brushfield's spots (gray or white spots around the edge of the iris), cataract.

eczema: Lid crusting, scaling, and oozing (blepharitis); conjunctivitis; conjunctival thickening; congestion of conjunctival blood vessels; dry eyes; keratoconus; cataract.

emphysema: Cataract (secondary to corticosteroid treatment).

endocarditis: Nystagmus, tiny red dots on conjunctiva, anisocoria, iritis.

facial deformity syndromes: Microphthalmos, downsloping lid slant, nystagmus, lower lid coloboma, dermoid cysts of the globe, cataract.

German measles (congenital defects following maternal infection): Microphthalmos, nystagmus, corneal edema, corneal clouding, iris atrophy, aniridia, cataract.

German measles (acute postnatal cases): Follicular conjunctivitis.

gonorrhea (neonatorum): Edema of orbit, lid edema, congestion of conjunctival blood vessels, conjunctival chemosis, purulent conjunctivitis, conjunctival pseudomembranes, keratitis, corneal perforation, iritis.

gout: Episcleritis, scleritis, corneal crystals, iritis.

hay fever: Conjunctivitis, congestion of conjunctival blood vessels, dry eye (secondary to medication), iritis (seasonal).

Herpes simplex (congenital defects following maternal infection): Cataract.

Herpes simplex (acute postnatal cases): Lid lesions, follicular conjunctivitis, limbal dendrites, corneal dendrites, corneal edema.

Herpes zoster: *See* shingles.

histoplasmosis: Conjunctivitis.

hypertension: Arcus senilis.

hypervitaminosis A, B, and D: Exophthalmos, calcium deposits in conjunctiva (D), band keratopathy (D), cataract (D).

influenza: Keratitis.

leprosy: Lash loss (brows and lids), paralysis of lid, thickened corneal nerves, corneal pannus, corneal scarring, corneal perforation, keratitis, iritis, iris nodules, cataract.

leukemia: Exophthalmos, metastatic lesions (visible mass, redness), symptoms of metastatic lesions (exophthalmos, hyphema).

lung cancer: Metastatic lesion to angle, metastatic lesion to iris, other metastatic lesions (visible mass, redness), symptoms of metastatic lesions (exophthalmos, hyphema).

lupus: Roundish lesions on lids, congestion of conjunctival blood vessels, episcleritis, keratitis, iridocyclitis.

malaria: Conjunctivitis, keratitis, iritis.

malnutrition: Lid edema, conjunctival chemosis, dry eye, keratopathy.

Marfan syndrome: Nystagmus, blue sclera, off-center pupil, multiple pupils, pupillary membrane, subluxed lens.

measles: Koplik's spots (tiny white grain surrounded by a red round area) on caruncle or conjunctiva, catarrhal conjunctivitis (inflammation with discharge), keratitis, iritis.

melanoma: Metastatic lesions (visible mass, redness), symptoms of metastatic lesions (exophthalmos, hyphema).

menopause: Increased wrinkling of skin, ectropion, entropion, ptosis, dermatochalasis, dry eye.

mononucleosis: Swelling indicating infection of the lacrimal gland, lid edema, conjunctivitis.

multiple sclerosis: Nystagmus, ptosis, anisocoria.

mumps: Swelling indicating infection of the lacrimal gland, conjunctivitis, episcleritis, scleritis, unilateral keratitis, stromal keratitis and vascularization (interstitial keratitis), iritis.

muscular dystrophy disorders: Ptosis, dry eye, cataract.

myasthenia gravis: Ptosis, abnormal pupil.

neurofibromatosis (von Recklinghausen's disease): Exophthalmos, thickened lid margins, lid neurofibroma, cafe-au-lait marks on lids, ptosis, limbal neurofibroma, prominent corneal nerves, iris nodules.

occlusive vascular disorder (progressive): Dilation of conjunctival vessels, iritis.

parathyroid (overactive): Calcification of conjunctiva, corneal opacities (calcium deposits), band keratopathy.

parathyroid (underactive): Blepharospasm, conjunctivitis, keratitis, cataract.

Parkinson's disease: Eyelid tremors, diminished blinking.

peptic ulcer disease: Iritis.

psoriasis: Scaling lid skin, blepharitis, exfoliated scales in conjunctival sac, conjunctivitis, corneal infiltrates, corneal erosion, corneal vascularization.

rheumatoid arthritis: Conjunctivitis, dry eye, episcleritis, scleritis, scleral thinning, keratitis sicca, band keratopathy, corneal melting, iritis, cataract.

rosacea: Blepharitis, conjunctivitis, multiple chalazia, keratitis, corneal ulcers, corneal infiltrates, corneal pannus, iritis.

rubeola: *See* measles.

rubella: *See* German measles.

sarcoidosis: Swelling of lacrimal gland, sarcoid lid nodule, episcleral nodule, keratic precipitates, corneal edema, iritis.

scleroderma: Scarring of lid margin, keratitis, corneal ulceration, cataract.

shingles (Herpes zoster): Vesicles on lid, ptosis, lid edema, lid redness, incomplete lid closure, scleritis, keratitis, exposure keratitis, corneal edema, infiltrates, iritis.

sickle cell disease: Comma-shaped conjunctival vessels.

sinus problems: Conjunctivitis, congestion of conjunctival blood vessels, dry eye (secondary to medication), iritis (seasonal).

smallpox: Lid lesions, trichiasis, symblepharon (lid adheres to the globe), conjunctivitis, severe keratitis, leukoma (white corneal opacity), iritis, patchy iris atrophy, vitreous opacity.

smoking: Dry eye, cataract.

temporal (cranial) arteritis: Iritis.

temporal (giant cell) arteritis: Ptosis, iritis.

third nerve palsy (oculomotor nerve palsy): Ptosis, anisocoria.

thyroid (overactive): Exophthalmos, orbital puffiness, lid retraction, lid lag, incomplete lid closure, exposure keratitis, keratoconjunctivitis of superior limbus.

thyroid (underactive): Periorbital edema, loss of outer third of brows, lid edema, mild cortical lens opacities.

toxoplasmosis (congenital and acquired): Conjunctivitis, leukokoria ("white pupil"), vitreous haze.

tuberculosis: Scleritis, phlyctenular keratoconjunctivitis (tiny red pustules on conjunctiva and/or cornea).

vaccinia: Lid infection, cellulitis, lid vesicles, blepharitis, conjunctivitis, keratitis, corneal perforation, vitreous opacity.

varicella: *See* chickenpox.

variola: *See* smallpox.

vitamin A deficiency: Foamy patches on bulbar conjunctiva, conjunctival dryness, corneal dryness, corneal haze, corneal perforation.

vitamin B deficiency: Conjunctival dryness, corneal dryness.

vitamin C deficiency: Subconjunctival hemorrhage.

Reprinted with permission from Ledford J, Sanders V. *The Slit Lamp Primer.* Thorofare, NJ: SLACK Incorporated; 1998: 95-98.

Systemic Disorders and Their Effects On the Eye*

DISORDER	OCULAR COMPLICATIONS
I. Cardiovascular	
A. Atherosclerosis/ carotid artery disease	Retinal artery obstruction
B. Endocarditis	Conjunctival and retinal hemorrhage (Roth's spot) Infection Artery occlusion
C. Hypertension	Narrowing, twisting, and fibrosis of retinal blood vessels Retinal hemorrhage Papilledema Cotton-wool spots
D. Mitral valve prolapse	Retinal vessel occlusion
II. Endocrine	
A. Diabetes	Leaking and rupturing of retinal blood vessels Neovascularization of retinal vessels Iris rubeosis Retinal detachment Macular edema Increased incidence of glaucoma and cataract

DISORDER	**OCULAR COMPLICATIONS**
B. Graves' disease	Inflammation of extraocular muscles (EOMs) Corneal exposure Compression of optic nerve
C. Hypothyroid	Partial loss of eyebrows and eyelashes Keratoconus Cataracts Optic atrophy
D. Pituitary tumor	Visual field loss Optic atrophy Nerve palsy

III. Infections

A. AIDS	Swelling of retinal vessels Cotton-wool patches Kaposi's sarcoma of lids, conjunctiva, or orbit
B. Chlamydia	Trachoma
C. Herpes simplex 1	Corneal opacity
D. Influenza	Conjunctivitis Dacryoadenitis
E. Lyme disease	Conjunctivitis Periorbital edema Corneal infiltrates Uveitis Endophthalmitis

DISORDER	**OCULAR COMPLICATIONS**
F. Measles	Conjunctivitis Subconjunctival hemorrhage Superficial keratitis
G. Shingles (Herpes zoster)	Corneal and lid lesions Inflammation of conjunctiva, sclera, and uvea
H. Syphilis	Eyelid chancre Argyll Robertson pupil Swelling of optic disc Optic atrophy EOM weakness
I. Toxoplasmosis	Chorioretinitis
J. Tuberculosis	Ocular tubercles

IV. Connective tissue disease

A. Lupus	Scleritis Damage to lacrimal gland Optic neuritis Cotton-wool spots
B. Multiple sclerosis	Optic neuritis Paralysis of EOMs Nystagmus
C. Rheumatoid arthritis	Keratoconjunctivitis sicca Scleritis Episcleritis Uveitis (in juveniles)
D. Temporal arteritis	Ischemic optic neuritis Weakness of EOMs

DISORDER	OCULAR COMPLICATIONS
V. Muscle disorders	
A. Muscular dystrophy	Weakness of EOMs (causing diplopia) Weakness of levator muscle (causing ptosis)
B. Myasthenia gravis	Weakness of EOMs Ptosis
VI. Blood dyscrasias	
A. Anemia	Pale conjunctiva Retinal hemorrhage Cotton-wool spots and hard exudates
B. Leukemia	Optic nerve compression Elevated IOP
C. Sickle cell disease	Neovascularization Vitreous hemorrhage Retinal detachment Elevated intraocular pressure (IOP)
VII. Age-related disorders	
A. Elderly	Cataract Macular degeneration Dry eye Increased incidence of glaucoma Increased incidence of infection Presbyopia (first noticed around age 40) Loss of skin and muscle tone

DISORDER	**OCULAR COMPLICATIONS**
	(entropion, ectropion, dermatochalasis, EOM dysfunction, ptosis)
B. Prematurity	O_2 damage to retina Blocked development of retinal blood vessels Retinal detachment Retinal scarring

VIII. Environmental disorders

A. Alcoholism	Visual field defects Nerve palsies Optic atrophy Alcohol amblyopia Decreased color vision Cataracts
B. Child abuse	Retinal and vitreal hemorrhage Periorbital bruising and swelling Subconjunctival hemorrhage Orbital fractures Hyphema Dislocated lens Retinal detachment
C. Malnutrition	Night blindness Retinopathy Corneal ulceration/necrosis
D. Smoking	Chronic conjunctivitis Increased risk of nuclear sclerosis Increased risk of macular degeneration

DISORDER	**OCULAR COMPLICATIONS**
	Increased optic nerve damage in glaucoma
	Nystagmus
	Optic neuropathy
IX. Genetic disorders	
A. Albinism	Blue-gray to pink iris
	Nystagmus
	Decreased visual acuity
	Strabismus
	Photophobia
B. Down syndrome	Short, slanted palpebral fissures
	Epicanthal folds
	Strabismus
	Nystagmus
	Myopia
	Cataracts
	Keratoconus
	Brushfield's spots
X. Neoplastic disorders	
A. Cancer	Ocular metastasis (iris most common)
B. Non-Hodgkin's lymphoma	Proptosis
	Conjunctival growths
	Diplopia
	Lacrimal gland infiltration
XI. Other disorders/conditions	
A. Chronic obstructive pulmonary disease	Dilation of retinal vessels
	Retinal hemorrhage
	Darkening of blood vessels (conjunctiva and retina)

DISORDER	**OCULAR COMPLICATIONS**
B. Gout	Conjunctivitis
	Episcleritis
	Scleritis
	Elevated IOP
	Uric acid crystals (cornea or sclera)
C. Pregnancy	Minor refractive shifts
	Difficulty with accommodation
	Drop in IOP
	Mild ptosis
	Hyperpigmentation of lids
D. Sarcoidosis	Bilateral anterior uveitis
	Granulomas
	Optic neuritis
	Optic atrophy

* See also Appendix 8

Ophthalmic Drugs

Note: See numbered lists starting on p. 261 for further information. The following is a list of brand name drugs. Please consult each drug's literature for further information. Mention of specific products is not intended as an endorsement by the author or publisher. A few medications are listed twice; this is because the ingredients vary from the drop to the ointment form.

BRAND NAME	USE(S)	LIST NUMBER
5-fluorouracil	Glaucoma surgery (inhibits scarring)	1
Absorbotear	Preserved artificial lubricant	2
Acular	Nonsteroidal anti-inflammatory	3
Adsorbonac	Corneal edema	1
Akarpine	Glaucoma	4
AK-Beta	Glaucoma	4
AK-Chlor	Antibiotic	5
AK-Cide	Steroidal anti-inflammatory/antibacterial	6
AK-Con	Decongestant	7
AK-Dex	Steroidal anti-inflammatory	3
AK-Dilate	Mydriasis	1
AK-Fluor	Dye study of fundus/iris	1

Brand Name	Use(s)	List Number
AK-NACL	Corneal edema	1
AK-Neo-Dex	Steroidal anti-inflammatory/antibiotic	6
AK-Nephrin	Decongestant	7
AK-Pentolate	Cycloplegia	1
AK-Poly-Bac	Antibiotic	5
AK-Pred	Steroidal anti-inflammatory	3
AK-Pro	Glaucoma	4
AK-Rinse	Irrigating solution	
AK-Spore HC	Steroidal anti-inflammatory/antibiotic	6
AK-Spore	Antibiotic	5
AK-Sulf	Antibacterial	5
AK-Taine	Anesthetic	1
AK-Tob	Antibiotic	5
AK-Tracin	Antibiotic	5
AK-Trol	Steroidal anti-inflammatory/antibiotic	6
Akwa Tears	Preserved artificial lubricant (drop)	2
Akwa Tears	Nonpreserved artificial lubricant (ointment)	2
Alamast	Mast cell stabilizer	8

Brand Name	Use(s)	List Number
Albalon	Decongestant	7
Alcaine	Anesthetic	1
All Clear	Decongestant/lubricant	7
All Clear AR	Decongestant/lubricant	7
Allerest	Decongestant	7
Alocril	Mast cell stabilizer	8
Alomide	Mast cell stabilizer	8
Alphagan	Glaucoma	4
Alrex	Steroidal anti-inflammatory	3
Amvisc Plus	Viscoelastic	1
Atropine Care	Cycloplegia	4
Azopt	Glaucoma	4
Betagan	Glaucoma	4
Betaxon	Glaucoma	4
Betimol	Glaucoma	4
Betoptic	Glaucoma	4
Betoptic-S	Glaucoma	4
BioLon	Viscoelastic	4
Bion Tears	Nonpreserved artificial lubricant	2

Brand Name	Use(s)	List Number
Bleph-10	Antibacterial	5
Blephamide	Steroidal anti-inflammatory/antibacterial	6
Blephamide SOP	Steroidal anti-inflammatory/antibacterial	6
Blinx	Irrigating solution	1
Botox	Muscle relaxant	4
Carbastat	Glaucoma	1
Cardio-green	Angiographic study	4
Carteolol	Glaucoma	2
Celluvisc	Nonpreserved artificial lubricant	5
Cetamide	Antibacterial	6
Cetapred	Steroidal anti-inflammatory/antibacterial	5
Chibroxin	Antibiotic	5
Chloromycetin	Antibiotic	5
Chloroptic	Antibiotic	5
Ciloxin	Antibiotic	7
Clarine	Decongestant	7
Clear Eyes	Decongestant/lubricant	7
Clear Eyes ACR	Decongestant/astringent	7
Collyrium	Irrigating solution	

Brand Name	Use(s)	List Number
Cortimycin	Steroidal anti-inflammatory/antibiotic	6
Cortisporin	Steroidal anti-inflammatory/antibiotic	6
Cosopt	Glaucoma	4
Crolom	Mast cell stabilizer	8
Cyclogyl	Cycloplegia	1
Cyclomydril	Cycloplegia/mydriasis	1
Dacriose	Irrigating solution	
Daranide	Glaucoma	4
Decadron	Steroidal anti-inflammatory	3
Dexacidin	Steroidal anti-inflammatory/antibiotic	6
Dexasol	Steroidal anti-inflammatory	3
Diamox	Glaucoma	4
Dry Eye Therapy	Nonpreserved artificial lubricant	2
Duolube	Nonpreserved artificial lubricant	2
Dura Tears Naturale	Preserved artificial lubricant	2
Duralube	Preserved artificial lubricant	2
Econopred	Steroidal anti-inflammatory	3
Econopred Plus	Steroidal anti-inflammatory	3
Eflone	Steroidal anti-inflammatory	3

Brand Name	Use(s)	List Number
Emadine	Antihistamine	8
Epifrin	Glaucoma	4
E-Pilo	Glaucoma	4
Epinal	Glaucoma	4
Eppy/N	Glaucoma	4
Eye-Sine	Decongestant	7
Eye Stream	Irrigating solution	
Eye Wash	Irrigating solution	
Flarex	Steroidal anti-inflammatory	3
Fluoracaine	Anesthetic/stain	1
Fluorescite	Dye study of fundus/iris	1
Fluor-op	Steroidal anti-inflammatory	3
Fluress	Anesthetic/stain	1
FML Forte	Steroidal anti-inflammatory	3
FML-S	Steroidal anti-inflammatory/antibacterial	6
FML SOP	Steroidal anti-inflammatory	3
Garamycin	Antibiotic	5
Geneyes	Decongestant	7
Genoptic	Antibiotic	5

Brand Name	Use(s)	List Number
Gentacidin	Antibiotic	5
Gentak	Antibiotic	5
GenTeal	Preserved artificial lubricant	2
GenTeal Gel	Preserved artificial lubricant	2
Glaucon	Glaucoma	4
Gonak	Coupling agent applied to diagnostic lens	1
Goniosol	Coupling agent applied to diagnostic lens	1
Healon	Viscoelastic	
Healon GV	Viscoelastic	
Herplex	Antiviral	5
HMS	Steroidal anti-inflammatory	3
Homatropine	Cycloplegia	1
Humorsol	Glaucoma	4
Hypotears	Preserved artificial lubricant	2
Hypotears PF	Nonpreserved artificial lubricant	2
IC-Green	Angiographic study	1
Ilotycin	Antibiotic	5
Inflamase Forte	Steroidal anti-inflammatory	3
Inflamase Mild	Steroidal anti-inflammatory	3

Brand Name	Use(s)	List Number
Iopidine	Glaucoma	4
Isopto Carbachol	Glaucoma	4
Isopto Carpine	Glaucoma	4
Isopto Cetamide	Antibacterial	5
Isopto Cetapred	Steroidal anti-inflammatory/antibacterial	6
Isopto-Hyoscine	Cycloplegia	1
Lacri-Gel	Nonpreserved artificial lubricant	2
Lacrilube NP	Nonpreserved artificial lubricant	2
Lacrilube SOP	Preserved artificial lubricant	2
Lacrisert	Artificial lubricant	2
Lipo-Tears	Nonpreserved artificial lubricant	2
Liquifilm	Steroidal anti-inflammatory	3
Liquifilm Tears	Preserved artificial lubricant	2
Livostin	Antihistamine	8
Lotemax	Steroidal anti-inflammatory	3
Lumigan	Glaucoma	4
Maxidex	Steroidal anti-inflammatory	3
Maxitrol	Steroidal anti-inflammatory/antibiotic	6
Metimyd	Steroidal anti-inflammatory/antibacterial	6

Brand Name	Use(s)	List Number
Miochol-E	Rapid miosis during surgery	1
Miostat	Rapid miosis during surgery	1
Moisture Eyes	Preserved artificial lubricant	2
Murine Tears	Preserved artificial lubricant	2
Murine Tears Plus	Decongestant/lubricant	7
Muro-128	Corneal edema	1
Mutamycin	Glaucoma surgery (inhibits scarring)	1
Mydfrin	Mydriasis	1
Mydriacyl	Cycloplegia	1
Napha-Forte	Decongestant	7
Naphcon	Decongestant	7
Naphcon-A	Decongestant/antihistamine	7
Natacyn	Antifungal	5
NeoDecadron	Steroidal anti-inflammatory/antibiotic	6
Neodexasone	Steroidal anti-inflammatory/antibiotic	6
Neopolydex	Steroidal anti-inflammatory/antibiotic	6
Neosporin	Antibiotic	5
Neo-Synephrine	Mydriasis	1

Brand Name	Use(s)	List Number
Neptazane	Glaucoma	4
Nutra-Tears	Preserved artificial lubricant	2
Ocuclear	Decongestant	7
Ocucoat	Preserved artificial lubricant	2
Ocucoat	Viscoelastic	3
Ocufen	Nonsteroidal anti-inflammatory	5
Ocuflox	Antibiotic	1
Oculinum	Muscle relaxant	4
Ocupress	Glaucoma	4
Ocusert	Glaucoma	7, 8
Opcon-A	Antihistamine/decongestant	1
Ophthaine	Anesthetic	1
Ophthetic	Anesthetic	6
Ophthocort	Steroidal anti-inflammatory/antibiotic	7
Opti-Clear	Decongestant	8
Opticrom	Mast cell stabilizer	7
Optigene 3	Decongestant	4
OptiPranolol	Glaucoma	4
P#E$_1$	Glaucoma	

Brand Name	Use(s)	List Number
Paremyd	Mydriasis	1
Patanol	Antihistamine	8
Phospholine iodide	Glaucoma	4
Pilagan	Glaucoma	4
Pilocar	Glaucoma	4
Pilopine	Glaucoma	4
Piloptic	Glaucoma	4
Pilostat	Glaucoma	4
Polymycin	Antibiotic	5
Poly-Pred	Steroidal anti-inflammatory/antibiotic	6
Polysporin	Antibiotic	5
Polytracin	Antibiotic	5
Polytrim	Antibiotic	5
Pontocaine	Anesthetic	1
Pred Forte	Steroidal anti-inflammatory	3
Pred G	Steroidal anti-inflammatory/antibiotic	6
Pred G SOP	Steroidal anti-inflammatory/antibiotic	6
Pred Mild	Steroidal anti-inflammatory	3
Pred-Phosphate	Steroidal anti-inflammatory	3

Brand Name	Use(s)	List Number
Profenal	Nonsteroidal anti-inflammatory	3
Propine	Glaucoma	4
ProVisc	Viscoelastic	5
Quixin	Antibacterial	2
Refresh	Preserved artificial lubricant	2
Refresh Plus	Nonpreserved artificial lubricant	2
Refresh PM	Nonpreserved artificial lubricant	4
Rescula	Glaucoma	1
Rev-Eyes	Reverse mydriasis	5
Sulamyd	Antibacterial	5
Sulf-10	Antibacterial	6
Sulfamide	Steroidal anti-inflammatory/antibacterial	2
Tears Naturale Free	Nonpreserved artificial lubricant	2
Tears Naturale II	Preserved artificial lubricant	1
Tensilon	Diagnosis of myasthenia gravis	5
TERAK	Antibiotic	5
Terramycin	Antibiotic	7
Tetrasine	Decongestant	4
Timoptic	Glaucoma	

Brand Name	Use(s)	List Number
Timoptic XE	Glaucoma	4
Tobradex	Steroidal anti-inflammatory/antibiotic	6
Tobralcon	Antibiotic	5
Tobrex	Antibiotic	5
Tomycine	Antibiotic	5
Travatan	Glaucoma	4
Tropicacyl	Cycloplegia	1
Trusopt	Glaucoma	4
Ultratears	Preserved artificial lubricant	2
Vasocidin	Steroidal anti-inflammatory/antibacterial	6
Vasocine	Steroidal anti-inflammatory/antibacterial	6
Vasoclear	Decongestant	7
Vasoclear-A	Decongestant/astringent	7
Vasocon-A	Decongestant/antihistamine	7, 8
Vexol	Steroidal anti-inflammatory	3
Vira-A	Antiviral	5
Viroptic	Antiviral	5
Viscoat	Viscoelastic	
Visine	Decongestant	7

Brand Name	Use(s)	List Number
Visine-A	Decongestant/antihistamine	7, 8
Visine AC	Decongestant/astringent	7
Visine LR	Decongestant	7
Visine Tears	Preserved artificial lubricant	2
Visine Tears PF	Nonpreserved artificial lubricant	2
Visudyne	Photodynamic therapy	1
Vit-A-Drops	Preserved artificial lubricant	2
Vitrasert	Antiviral	5
Vitravene	Antiviral	5
Vitraz	Viscoelastic	
Voltaren	Nonsteroidal anti-inflammatory	3
Xalatan	Glaucoma	4
Zacril	Preserved artificial lubricant	2
Zaditor	Mast cell stabilizer/antihistamine	8
Zincfrin	Decongestant/astringent	7

LIST 1

Diagnostics/Miscellaneous

Note: All drugs are in topical drop form unless otherwise noted

BRAND NAME	GENERIC NAME	USE
5-fluorouracil	Fluorouracil (injection)	Glaucoma surgery
Adsorbonac	Sodium chloride (gtt/ung)	Corneal edema
AK-Dilate	Phenylephrine	Mydriasis
AK-Fluor	Fluorescein (injection)	Dye study of fundus/iris
AK-NACL	Sodium chloride (gtt/ung)	Corneal edema
AK-Pentolate	Cyclopentolate	Cycloplegia
AK-Taine	Proparacaine	Anesthetic
Alcaine	Proparacaine	Anesthetic
Atropine Care	Atropine	Cycloplegia
Botox	Botulinum toxin type A (injection)	Muscle relaxant
Cardio-green	Indocyanine green (injection)	Angiographic study
Cyclogyl	Cyclopentolate	Cycloplegia
Cyclomydril	Cyclopentolate/phenylephrine	Cycloplegia/mydriasis

Brand Name	Generic Name	Use
Fluoracaine	Proparacaine/fluorescein	Anesthetic/stain
Fluorescite	Fluorescein (injection)	Dye study of fundus/iris
Fluress	Benoxinate/fluorescein	Anesthetic/stain
Gonak	Methylcellulose	Coupling agent applied to diagnostic lens
Goniosol	Methylcellulose	Coupling agent applied to diagnostic lens
Homatropine	Homatropine	Cycloplegia
IC-Green	Indocyanine green (injection)	Angiographic study
Isopto-Hyoscine	Scopolamine	Cycloplegia
Miochol-E	Acetylcholine (intraocular)	Rapid miosis during surgery
Miostat	Carbachol (intraocular)	Rapid miosis during surgery
Muro-128	Sodium chloride (gtt/ung)	Corneal edema
Mutamycin	Mitomycin C (injection)	Glaucoma surgery (inhibits scarring)
Mydfrin	Phenylephrine	Mydriasis
Mydriacyl	Tropicamide	Cycloplegia
Neo-Synephrine	Phenylephrine	Mydriasis
Oculinum	Botulinum toxin type A (injection)	Muscle relaxant
Ophthaine	Proparacaine	Anesthetic

Brand Name	Generic Name	Use
Ophthetic	Proparacaine	Anesthetic
Paremyd	Hydroxyamphetamine	Mydriasis
Pontocaine	Tetracaine	Anesthetic
Rev-Eyes	Dapiprazole	Reverse mydriasis
Tensilon	Edrophonium	Diagnosis of myasthenia gravis
Tropicacyl	Tropicamide	Cycloplegia
Visudyne	Verteporfin	Photodynamic therapy

gtt = drop; ung = ointment

LIST 2

Artificial Ocular Lubricants

BRAND NAME	TYPE OF LUBRICANT	FORM
Absorbotear	Preserved	Drops
Akwa Tears	Preserved	Drops
Akwa Tears	Nonpreserved	Ointment
Bion Tears	Nonpreserved	Drops
Celluvisc	Nonpreserved	Drops
Dry Eye Therapy	Nonpreserved	Drops
Duolube	Nonpreserved	Ointment
Dura Tears Naturale	Nonpreserved	Ointment
Duralube	Preserved	Ointment
GenTeal	Preserved	Drops
GenTeal Gel	Preserved	Gel
Hypotears	Preserved	Drops, ointment
Hypotears PF	Nonpreserved	Drops
Lacri-Gel	Nonpreserved	Gel

Brand Name	Type of Lubricant	Form
Lacrilube NP	Nonpreserved	Ointment
Lacrilube SOP	Preserved	Ointment
Lacrisert	N/A	Pellet
Lipo-Tears	Nonpreserved	Ointment
Liquifilm Tears	Preserved	Drops
Moisture Eyes	Preserved	Ointment
Murine Tears	Preserved	Drops
Nutra-Tears	Preserved	Drops
Ocucoat	Preserved	Drops
Refresh	Preserved	Drops
Refresh Plus	Nonpreserved	Drops
Refresh PM	Nonpreserved	Ointment
Tears Naturale Free	Nonpreserved	Drops
Tears Naturale II	Preserved	Drops
Ultratears	Preserved	Drops
Visine Tears	Preserved	Drops
Visine Tears PF	Nonpreserved	Drops
Vit-A-Drops	Preserved	Drops
Zacril	Preserved	Drops

List 3

Anti-Inflammatories

Brand Name	Generic Name	Type
Acular	Ketorolac	NSAID
AK-Dex	Dexamethasone	Steroid/anti-inflammatory
AK-Pred	Prednisolone	Steroid/anti-inflammatory
Alrex	Loteprednol	Steroid/anti-inflammatory
Decadron	Dexamethasone	Steroid/anti-inflammatory
Dexasol	Dexamethasone	Steroid/anti-inflammatory
Econopred	Prednisolone	Steroid/anti-inflammatory
Econopred Plus	Prednisolone	Steroid/anti-inflammatory
Eflone	Fluorometholone	Steroid/anti-inflammatory
Flarex	Fluorometholone	Steroid/anti-inflammatory
Fluor-op	Fluorometholone	Steroid/anti-inflammatory
FML Forte	Fluorometholone	Steroid/anti-inflammatory
FML SOP	Fluorometholone	Steroid/anti-inflammatory

Brand Name	Generic Name	Type
HMS	Medrysone	Steroid/anti-inflammatory
Inflamase Forte	Prednisolone	Steroid/anti-inflammatory
Inflamase Mild	Prednisolone	Steroid/anti-inflammatory
Liquifilm	Fluorometholone	Steroid/anti-inflammatory
Lotemax	Loteprednol	Steroid/anti-inflammatory
Maxidex	Dexamethasone	Steroid/anti-inflammatory
Ocufen	Flurbiprofen	NSAID
Pred Forte	Prednisolone	Steroid/anti-inflammatory
Pred Mild	Prednisolone	Steroid/anti-inflammatory
Pred-Phosphate	Prednisolone	Steroid/anti-inflammatory
Profenal	Suprofen	NSAID
Vexol	Rimexolone	Steroid/anti-inflammatory
Voltaren	Diclofenac	NSAID

NSAID = nonsteroidal anti-inflammatory drug

LIST 4

Glaucoma Medications

BRAND NAME	GENERIC	CLASS
Akarpine	Pilocarpine	Miotic
AK-Beta	Levobunolol	Nonselective β blocker
AK-Pro	Dipivefrin	α,β adrenergic agonist
Alphagan	Brimonidine	Pure α-2 adrenergic agonist
Azopt	Brinzolamide	CAI
Betagan	Levobunolol	Nonselective β blocker
Betaxon	Levobetaxolol	Selective β-1 blocker
Betimol	Timolol	Nonselective β blocker
Betoptic	Betaxolol	Selective β-1 blocker
Betoptic-S	Betaxolol suspension	Selective β-1 blocker
Carbastat	Carbachol	Miotic
Carteolol	Carteolol	Nonselective β blocker
Cosopt	Timolol/dorzolamide	Nonselective β blocker/CAI

Brand Name	Generic	Class
Daranide	Dichlorphenamide oral	CAI
Diamox	Acetazolamide oral	CAI
Epifrin	Epinephrine	α,β adrenergic agonist
E-Pilo	Pilocarpine/epinephrine	Miotic/α,β adrenergic agonist
Epinal	Epinephrine	α,β adrenergic agonist
Eppy/N	Epinephrine	α,β adrenergic agonist
Glaucon	Epinephrine	α,β adrenergic agonist
Humorsol	Demecarium	Miotic
Iopidine	Apraclonidine	Pure α-2 adrenergic agonist
Isopto Carbachol	Carbachol	Miotic
Isopto Carpine	Pilocarpine	Miotic
Lumigan	Bimatoprost	Prostaglandin
Neptazane	Methazolamide oral	CAI
Ocupress	Carteolol	Nonselective β blocker
Ocusert	Pilocarpine insert	Miotic
OptiPranolol	Metipranolol	Nonselective β blocker
P#E$_1$	Pilocarpine/epinephrine	Miotic/α,β adrenergic agonist
Phospholine iodide	Echothiophate	Miotic
Pilagan	Pilocarpine	Miotic

Brand Name	Generic	Class
Pilocar	Pilocarpine	Miotic
Pilopine	Pilocarpine gel	Miotic
Piloptic	Pilocarpine	Miotic
Pilostat	Pilocarpine	Miotic
Propine	Dipivefrin	α,β adrenergic agonist
Rescula	Unoprostone	Currently unknown
Timoptic	Timolol	Nonselective β blocker
Timoptic XE	Timolol gel	Nonselective β blocker
Travatan	Travoprost	Prostaglandin
Trusopt	Dorzolamide	CAI
Xalatan	Latanoprost	Prostaglandin

α =alpha; β = beta; CAI = carbonic anhydrase inhibitor

Anti-Infectives

LIST 5

BRAND NAME	INGREDIENT(S)	USE	FORM(S)
AK-Chlor	Chloramphenicol	Antibiotic	gtt
AK-Poly-Bac	Polymixin/bacitracin	Antibiotic	ung
AK-Spore	Polymixin B/neomycin/gramicidin	Antibiotic	gtt/ung
AK-Spore	Polymixin B/neomycin/bacitracin	Antibiotic	ung
AK-Sulf	Sulfacetamide	Antibacterial	gtt/ung
AK-Tob	Tobramycin	Antibiotic	gtt
AK-Tracin	Bacitracin	Antibiotic	gtt/ung
Bleph-10	Sulfacetamide	Antibacterial	gtt/ung
Cetamide	Sulfacetamide	Antibacterial	ung
Chibroxin	Norfloxacin	Antibiotic	gtt
Chloromycetin	Chloramphenicol	Antibiotic	gtt/ung
Chloroptic	Chloramphenicol	Antibiotic	gtt/ung
Ciloxin	Ciprofloxacin	Antibiotic	gtt/ung
Garamycin	Gentamicin	Antibiotic	gtt/ung

Brand Name	Ingredient(s)	Use	Form(s)
Genoptic	Gentamicin	Antibiotic	gtt/ung
Gentacidin	Gentamicin	Antibiotic	gtt/ung
Gentak	Gentamicin	Antibiotic	gtt/ung
Herplex	Idoxuridine	Antiviral	gtt
Ilotycin	Erythromycin	Antibiotic	ung
Isopto Cetamide	Sulfacetamide	Antibacterial	gtt
Natacyn	Natamycin	Antifungal	gtt
Neosporin	Polymixin B/neomycin/bacitracin	Antibiotic	gtt/ung
Neosporin	Polymixin B/neomycin/gramicidin	Antibiotic	gtt
Ocuflox	Ofloxacin	Antibiotic	gtt
Polymycin	Polymixin B/neomycin/gramicidin	Antibiotic	gtt/ung
Polysporin	Polymixin/bacitracin	Antibiotic	ung
Polytracin	Polymixin/bacitracin	Antibiotic	ung
Polytrim	Polymixin B/trimethoprim	Antibiotic	gtt
Quixin	Levofloxacin	Antibiotic	gtt
Sulamyd	Sulfacetamide	Antibacterial	gtt/ung
Sulf-10	Sulfacetamide	Antibacterial	gtt
TERAK	Polymixin B/oxytetracycline	Antibiotic	ung
Terramycin	Polymixin B/oxytetracycline	Antibiotic	ung

Brand Name	Ingredient(s)	Use	Form(s)
Tobralcon	Tobramycin	Antibiotic	gtt/ung
Tobrex	Tobramycin	Antibiotic	ung
Tomycine	Tobramycin	Antibiotic	gtt
Vira-A	Vidarabine	Antiviral	gtt
Viroptic	Trifluridine	Antiviral	gtt
Vitrasert	Ganciclovir	Antiviral	implant
Vitravene	Fomivirsen	Antiviral	vitreous inj

gtt = drop; ung = ointment; inj = injection

LIST 6

Anti-Infective/Anti-Inflammatory Combinations

BRAND NAME	INGREDIENTS	USE	FORM(S)
AK-Cide	Sulfacetamide/prednisolone	ster/slf	gtt/ung
AK-Neo-Dex	Neomycin/dexamethasone	ster/antib	gtt/ung
AK-Spore HC	Bacitracin/neomycin/polymixin B/hydrocortisone	ster/antib	ung
AK-Spore HC	Neomycin/polymixin B/hydrocortisone	ster/antib	gtt
AK-Trol	Neomycin/polymixin B/dexamethasone	ster/antib	gtt/ung
Blephamide	Sulfacetamide/prednisolone	ster/slf	gtt/ung
Blephamide SOP	Sulfacetamide/prednisolone	ster/slf	ung
Cetapred	Sulfacetamide/prednisolone	ster/slf	gtt/ung
Cortimycin	Neomycin/polymixin B/hydrocortisone	ster/antib	gtt/ung
Cortisporin	Bacitracin/neomycin/polymixin B/hydrocortisone	ster/antib	ung
Cortisporin	Neomycin/polymixin B/hydrocortisone	ster/antib	gtt
Dexacidin	Neomycin/polymixin B/dexamethasone	ster/antib	gtt/ung
FML-S	Sulfacetamide/fluorometholone	ster/slf	gtt

Brand Name	Ingredients	Use	Form(s)
Isopto Cetapred	Sulfacetamide/prednisolone	ster/slf	gtt
Maxitrol	Neomycin/polymixin B/dexamethasone	ster/antib	gtt/ung
Metimyd	Sulfacetamide/prednisolone	ster/slf	gtt/ung
NeoDecadron	Neomycin/dexamethasone	ster/antib	gtt/ung
Neodexasone	Neomycin/dexamethasone	ster/antib	gtt
Neopolydex	Neomycin/polymixin B/dexamethasone	ster/antib	gtt/ung
Ophthocort	Chloramphenicol/polymixin B/hydrocortisone	ster/antib	ung
Poly-Pred	Neomycin/polymixin B/prednisolone	ster/antib	gtt
Pred G	Gentamicin/prednisolone	ster/antib	gtt
Pred G SOP	Prednisolone acetate/gentamicin	ster/antib	ung
Sulfamide	Sulfacetamide/prednisolone	ster/slf	gtt/ung
Tobradex	Tobramycin/dexamethasone	ster/antib	gtt/ung
Vasocidin	Sulfacetamide/prednisolone	ster/slf	gtt/ung
Vasocine	Sulfacetamide/prednisolone	ster/slf	ung

ster = steroid; slf = sulfonamide; antib = antibiotic; gtt = drop; ung = ointment

LIST 7

Decongestants/Combinations

BRAND NAME	GENERIC NAME/ACTIVE INGREDIENT(S)	USE(S)
AK-Con	Naphazoline	Decongestant
AK-Nephrin	Phenylephrine	Decongestant
Albalon	Naphazoline	Decongestant
All Clear	Naphazoline/polyethylene glycol	Decongestant/lubricant
All Clear AR	Naphazoline/methyl cellulose	Decongestant/lubricant
Allerest	Naphazoline	Decongestant
Clarine	Tetrahydrozoline	Decongestant
Clear Eyes	Naphazoline/glycerin	Decongestant/lubricant
Clear Eyes ACR	Naphazoline/zinc/glycerin	Decongestant/astringent
Eye-Sine	Tetrahydrozoline	Decongestant
Geneyes	Tetrahydrozoline	Decongestant
Murine Tears Plus	Tetrahydrozoline/polyvinyl alcohol/povidone	Decongestant/lubricant
Napha-Forte	Naphazoline	Decongestant

BRAND NAME	GENERIC NAME/ACTIVE INGREDIENT(S)	USE(S)
Naphcon	Naphazoline	Decongestant
Naphcon-A	Naphazoline/pheniramine maleate	Decongestant/antihistamine
Ocuclear	Oxymetazoline	Decongestant
Opcon-A	Naphazoline/pheniramine maleate	Decongestant/antihistamine
Opti-Clear	Tetrahydrozoline	Decongestant
Optigene 3	Tetrahydrozoline	Decongestant
Tetrasine	Tetrahydrozoline	Decongestant
Vasoclear	Naphazoline	Decongestant
Vasoclear-A	Naphazoline/zinc	Decongestant/astringent
Vasocon-A	Naphazoline/antazoline	Decongestant/antihistamine
Visine	Tetrahydrozoline	Decongestant
Visine-A	Naphazoline/pheniramine maleate	Decongestant/antihistamine
Visine AC	Tetrahydrozoline/zinc sulfate	Decongestant/astringent
Visine LR	Oxymetazoline	Decongestant
Zincfrin	Phenylephrine/zinc	Decongestant/astringent

List 8

Anti-Allergenics

Brand Name	Ingredients	Type
Alamast	Pemirolast	MCS
Alocril	Nedocromil	MCS
Alomide	Lodoxamide	MCS
Crolom	Cromolyn	MCS
Emadine	Emedastine	antihis
Livostin	Levocabastine	antihis
Opcon-A	Pheneramine/naphazoline	antihis/decon
Opticrom	Cromolyn	MCS
Patanol	Olopatadine	antihis
Vasocon-A	Antazoline/naphazoline	antihis/decon
Visine-A	Pheneramine/naphazoline	antihis/decon
Zaditor	Ketotifen	MCS/antihis

MCS = mast cell stabilizer; antihis = antihistamine; decon = decongestant

Lasers in Ophthalmology

LASER	WAVELENGTH	ACTION	USES
I. Thermal Argon	Blue-green (488 to 515 nm) Low energy Continuous wave	Photocoagulation Absorbed by hemoglobin, melanin, and xanthophyll	Retinal vascular disease Choroidal neovascularization Trabeculoplasty Iridotomy Suture lysis
Krypton	Red (647 nm) Continuous wave	Photocoagulation Absorbed by melanin, to a lesser degree by hemoglobin (not absorbed by retinal vessels and xanthophyll) Passes more readily through lens opacities and vitreous hemorrhages	Same as argon but deeper choroid

LASER	WAVELENGTH	ACTION	USES
CO_2	Infrared Long wavelength Low penetration	Photovaporization (photo-evaporation) Absorbed by water	Skin lesions Fine, bloodless skin incisions Cautery
Tunable dye	Adjustable (green to red)	Photocoagulation Variably absorbed by melanin, hemoglobin, and xanthophyll	Same as argon and krypton
Diode laser	Infrared (805 nm)	Photocoagulation Sometimes used in conjunction with ICG dye	Retinal vascular disease Choroidal neovascularization
Frequency-doubled YAG	Green (532 nm) Continuous wave	Photocoagulation	Same as krypton

LASER	WAVELENGTH	ACTION	USES
II. Ionizing Q-switched YAG	Infrared (1064 nm) Pulsed laser	Photodisruption (cold, cutting) Very tiny spot sizes	Incisions/cutting Synechotomy Capsulotomy Vitreous adhesions Iridotomy
III. Photochemical Excimer	UV light (photo-evaporation)	Photoablation Breaks chemical bonds of tissues	Corneal opacities Refractive surgery
Photodynamic therapy	Red-infrared (665 to 732 nm)	Causes chemical changes that result in vascular occlusion and cellular disruption Used in conjunction with photosensitive agents	Malignant tumors Choroidal neovascularization

Reprinted with permission from Ledford J. *Certified Ophthalmic Medical Technologist Exam Review Manual.* Thorofare, NJ: SLACK Incorporated; 2000.

Ocular and Systemic Effects of Topical Ocular Drugs

DRUG TYPE	OCULAR	SYSTEMIC
Decongestant	Increased redness Dryness Pupil dilation Transient stinging	Nervousness Decreased heart rate Headache, nervousness
Corticosteroids	PSC cataract Elevated IOP (no symptoms)	Stomach ulcers Psychoses Muscle weakness Bone weakness
NSAIDs	Transient stinging Follicular conjunctivitis	Stomach upset Stomach ulcers Vomiting Promote asthma

Drug Type	Ocular	Systemic
Antibiotics	Transient stinging Allergic reaction Redness Photophobia Depigmentation of eyelids	Dermatitis Digestive upset
Antivirals	Transient stinging Corneal toxicity	Contact dermatitis
Direct-acting adrenergics	Transient stinging Redness	Arousal of sympathetic nervous system
Beta blockers	Transient stinging	Decreased heart rate Slowed breathing Depression Confusion Dizziness Digestive upset Headache

Drug Type	Ocular	Systemic
Beta blockers (continued)		Rash Insomnia Impotence Decreased appetite
Miotics	Transient stinging Blurred vision Miosis Accommodative spasm Posterior synechiae	Brow headache Sweating Salivation Digestive upset Decreased heart rate Flushing Tremors Difficulty breathing Lethargy
Carbonic anhydrase inhibitors	Conjunctival irritation	Bitter taste

Reprinted with permission from Ledford J. *The Complete Guide to Ocular History Taking.* Thorofare, NJ: SLACK Incorporated; 1999: 42.

Normal Values of Common Blood Tests

1. Complete blood count (CBC)—Checks the number of red blood cells, white blood cells, and platelets present in a blood sample. Normal values are:
    White blood cell count: 4300 to 10,800/cu mm
    Platelet count: 150,000 to 350,000/cu mm
    Red cell count:
        Male: 4.6 to 6.2 million/cu mm
        Female: 4.2 to 5.4 million/cu mm
    Hemoglobin:
        Male: 14 to 17 g/dL
        Female: 12 to 15 g/dL
    Hematocrit:
        Male: 41% to 50%
        Female: 36% to 44%

2. Prothrombin time—Evaluates the ability of the blood to clot. A normal value is between 9 and 18 seconds.

3. Blood glucose level—Used to detect the presence of diabetes and to monitor its treatment. Normal fasting blood glucose level is 60 to 100 mg/dL.

4. Rheumatoid factor—A test for rheumatoid arthritis. If the patient does not have rheumatoid arthritis, the test will usually be negative.

5. Erythrocyte sedimentation rate—Indicates the presence and intensity of an inflammatory process such as arthritis or cancer. It is not specific for any one disease. Normal values (Westergren) are:

Male: 0 to 13 mm/hour
Female: 0 to 20 mm/hour

6. Creatinine and blood urea nitrogen (BUN)—Both creatinine and BUN are tests of kidney function. Normal values are:
    Creatinine: 0.8 to 1.2 mg/dL
    BUN: 8 to 25 mg/dL

7. Potassium—3.3 to 4.9 mmol/L

8. Sodium—135 to 145 mmol/L

9. Calcium—8.9 to 10.3 mg/dL

Note: Some normals vary slightly according to the patient's age, the laboratory, and the test manufacturer.

The Metric System

The metric system is a system for measuring length, weight, and volume. It is used in most English-speaking countries, although its acceptance in the United States has been slow.

The beauty of the metric system lies in the fact that it is based on multiples of 10. In addition, the same prefixes indicating fractions of units can be applied to all three types of measurements.

The base metric unit for length is the meter. The gram is the base for weight, and the liter for volume. *Metric Fraction Prefixes* (p. 290) shows the prefixes that are most useful in the eyecare field. These prefixes can be combined to any of the base units. For example, the terms kilometer, kilogram, and kiloliter all refer to 10^3 of their respective units (ie, 1000 m, gm, or l).

The metric system is widely used in the scientific community, including the eyecare field. Because of this, most of the formulas used in optics are written to use metric units. If your measurements are taken in nonmetric units (eg, inches, pounds, or fluid ounces), you will need to be able to convert them to metric units in order to work the formula. *Metric Equivalents* (p. 290) gives common conversions.

It is also important to note that while measurements may be given in the metric system, the formula may call for a different fraction unit. For example, the formula for focal length is $D = 1 \div F$ where D is the power of the lens in diopters and F is the focal length in meters. However, you may be given the focal length in centimeters. It is important to know the formula and to read the question carefully in order to be sure that you are working with the correct units. If not, it is easy to go from one unit to the other by moving the decimal point accordingly.

At times, it may also be necessary to be able to convert visual acuity measurements from those based on 20 feet to those based on the metric system (6 m is standard). *Visual Acuity Equivalents* (p. 291) gives these conversions.

METRIC FRACTION PREFIXES

Prefix	*Part of Base Unit*
Kilo	10^3 or base unit x 1000
Hecto	10^2 or base unit x 100
Deci	10^{-1} or base unit x 0.1
Centi	10^{-2} or base unit x 0.01
Milli	10^{-3} or base unit x 0.001
Micro	10^{-6} or base unit x 0.000001

Base units: meter (length), liter (liquid measurement), square meters (square measurement), gram (weight), and cubic meters (cubic measure).

METRIC EQUIVALENTS

1 centimeter	0.3937 inch (centimeters x 0.3937 = inches)
1 inch	2.54 centimeters (inches x 2.54 = centimeters)
1 meter	39.37 inches (meters x 39.37 = inches)
1 yard	0.9144 meter (yards x 0.9144 = meters)
1 cubic centimeter	0.061 inch^3 (cubic centimeters x 0.061 = inches^3)
1 cubic inch	16.39 cc (cubic inches x 16.39 = cc)

1 ounce	28.3 grams (ounces x 28.3 = grams)
1 liter	2.11 pints (liters x 2.11 = pints)
1 gallon	3.79 liters (gallons x 3.79 = liters)
1 gram	0.035 ounces (grams x 0.035 = ounces)
1 pound	28.3 grams (pounds x 28.3 = grams)
1 kilogram	2.2 pounds (kilograms x 2.2 = pounds)

VISUAL ACUITY EQUIVALENTS

Based on 20 Feet	*Based on 6 Meters*
20/400	6/120
20/300	6/90
20/200	6/60
20/100	6/30
20/80	6/24
20/70	6/21
20/60	6/18
20/50	6/15
20/40	6/12
20/30	6/9
20/25	6/7.5
20/20	6/6
20/15	6/4.5
20/10	6/3

Reprinted with permission from Lens A. *Optics, Retinoscopy, and Refractometry.* Thorofare, NJ: SLACK Incorporated; 1999: 72-73.

English and Metric Conversion

LINEAR MEASURE

1 centimeter = 0.3937 inch
1 inch = 2.54 centimeters
1 foot = 0.3048 meter
1 meter = 39.37 inches/1.0936 yards
1 yard = 0.9144 meter
1 kilometer = 0.621 mile
1 mile = 1.609 kilometers

SQUARE MEASURE

1 square centimeter = 0.1550 square inch
1 square inch = 6.452 square centimeters
1 square foot = 0.0929 square meter
1 square meter = 1.196 square yards
1 square yard = 0.8361 square meter
1 hectare = 2.47 acres
1 acre = 0.4047 hectare
1 square kilometer = 0.386 square mile
1 square mile = 2.59 square kilometers

WEIGHT MEASURE

1 gram = 0.03527 ounce
1 ounce = 28.35 grams
1 kilogram = 2.2046 pounds
1 pound = 0.4536 kilogram
1 metric ton = 0.98421 English ton
1 English ton = 1.016 metric tons

VOLUME MEASURE

1 cubic centimeter = 0.061 cubic inch
1 cubic inch = 16.39 cubic centimeters
1 cubic foot = 0.0283 cubic meter
1 cubic meter = 1.308 cubic yards
1 cubic yard = 0.7646 cubic meter
1 liter = 1.0567 quarts
1 quart dry = 1.101 liters
1 quart liquid = 0.9463 liter
1 gallon = 3.78541 liters
1 peck = 8.810 liters
1 hectoliter = 2.8375 bushels

Reprinted with permission from Jacobs K, Jacobs L. *Quick Reference Dictionary for Occupational Therapy.* 3rd ed. Thorofare, NJ: SLACK Incorporated; 2001: 445.

Weights and Measures

LINEAR MEASURE

12 inches = 1 foot
3 feet = 1 yard (0.9144 meter)
5.5 yards = 1 rod
40 rods = 1 furlong/220 yards
8 furlongs = 1 statute mile/1760 yards
5280 feet = 1 statute or land mile
3 miles = 1 league
6076.11549 feet = 1 international nautical mile (1852 meters)

DRY MEASURE

2 pints = 1 quart
8 quarts = 1 peck
4 pecks = 1 bushel/2150.42 cubic inches

ANGULAR AND CIRCULAR MEASURE

60 seconds = 1 minute
60 minutes = 1 degree
90 degrees = 1 right angle
180 degrees = 1 straight angle
360 degrees = 1 circle

SQUARE MEASURE

144 square inches = 1 square foot
9 square feet = 1 square yard
30.25 square yards = 1 square rod

160 square rods = 1 acre
640 acres = 1 square mile

TROY WEIGHT

24 grains = 1 pennyweight
20 pennyweights = 1 ounce
12 ounces = 1 pound, Troy

CUBIC MEASURE

1728 cubic inches = 1 cubic foot
27 cubic feet = 1 cubic yard

LIQUID MEASURE

4 gills = 1 pint
2 pints = 1 quart
4 quarts = 1 gallon/231.0 cubic inches

AVOIRDUPOIS WEIGHT

27.34375 grains = 1 dram
16 drams = 1 ounce
16 ounces = 1 pound/0.45359237 kilogram
100 pounds = 1 short hundredweight
20 short hundredweights = 1 short ton

Reprinted with permission from Jacobs K, Jacobs L. *Quick Reference Dictionary for Occupational Therapy.* 3rd ed. Thorofare, NJ: SLACK Incorporated; 2001: 441-442.

Manual Alphabet for Communicating With the Hearing Impaired

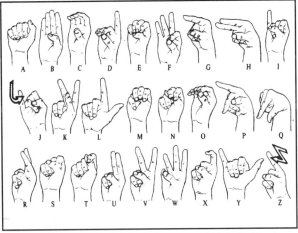

Reprinted with permission from the National Technical Institute for the Deaf, Rochester, NY.

The Braille Alphabet

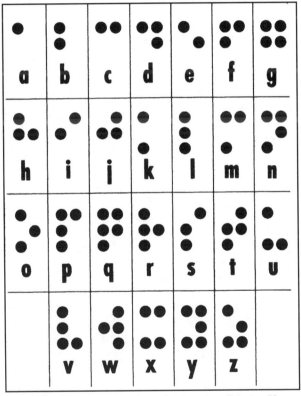

Reprinted with permission from the American Printing House for the Blind, Louisville, Ky.

Certification as Paraoptometric and Ophthalmic Medical Personnel

The eyecare field is vast. It provides many opportunities for motivated persons to advance themselves. Information given here is taken from the most recent data available prior to publication; contact your certifying body for the most current information.

PARAOPTOMETRY

The American Optometric Association, Paraoptometric Section, offers three levels of certification: certified paraoptometric (CPO), certified paraoptometric assistant (CPOA), and certified paraoptometric technician (CPOT). One must qualify to take the written exam at each level, and there are several options. First, for job-trained candidates, qualification is earned by working in the field; in addition, CPOA candidates must first earn the CPO rank, and CPOT candidates must hold current CPOA status. Alternately, candidates may qualify for the exams during their last semester in an optometric assistant or accredited technician program. Those passing the CPOT written exam must additionally pass a skills examination before the title is awarded.

Topics covered in the CPO exam are (as taken from the chapter headings of the study guide/workbook, which is sent to every registering CPO candidate) eyecare specialists and ancillary personnel, practice management and telephone techniques, anatomy of the eye, the eye examination, refractive status, the ophthalmic prescription (referring to lenses), ophthalmic lenses, ophthalmic dispensing, contact lenses, common eye disorders, and terminology.

Exam criteria for the CPOA includes practice management (office procedures, patient handling, office finances, professional issues), ophthalmic optics and dispensing (prescriptions, lenses, frame selection, adjustment, and dispensing), basic procedures (basic concepts and procedures for preliminary testing, visual acuity, color vision, stereo acuity, case history, familiarity with examination instrumentation), special procedures (contact lenses, tonometry, visual fields, sphygmomanometry, first aid, low vision), refractive status of the eye and binocularity (refractive errors, refractive conditions, terminology and definitions of eye movements, binocular vision), and basic ocular anatomy and physiology (location and definition of parts of the eye, basic functions, definitions and causes of common pathological and functional disorders, basic ocular pharmacology).

The written exam for CPOT covers pretesting procedures (case history, visual acuity, vision screening and preliminary testing techniques, color vision, stereo acuity), clinical procedures (keratometry, tonometry, visual fields, sphygmomanometry, contact lenses, vision therapy, triage/first aid, low vision, special ocular procedures), ophthalmic optics and dispensing (optical principles of light, prescriptions, lenses, frame selection, adjustment), refractive status of the eye and binocularity (refractive errors, refractive conditions, eye movements, binocular vision), anatomy and physiology (general anatomy and physiology of the eye), and practice management (office management, professional issues, government rules and regulations).

The CPOT practical exam utilizes five stations. Station 1 is case history. Station 2 is visual acuity, stereopsis, color vision, externals, ocular motility, pupil testing, pupillary distance (PD) measurement, and cover test.

Station 3 is ophthalmic dispensing (neutralization, verification, duplication). Station 4 is contact lenses (soft lens: preparation, insertion, removal; rigid lens: preparation, insertion, removal; hygiene). Station 5 is asepsis, patching, drop instillation, and blood pressure measurement.

For information on the home study course and to obtain a handbook for the examinations, contact:

American Optometric Association
Paraoptometric Section
243 N. Lindbergh Blvd.
St. Louis, MO 63141-7881
Phone: 1-800-365-2219 or 314-991-4100
Fax: 314-991-4101
E-mail: ps@theaoa.org

The American Optometric Association has put together a self-study course that is especially recommended (but not required) for those seeking certification at the CPOA level. Ordering information can be obtained at the address above. In addition to the home study course, there are other study materials available for those who wish to prepare for examinations. *The Basic Bookshelf for Eyecare Professionals* (a 24-book set published by SLACK Incorporated) was written to include all the exam content areas one needs to review for the tests. Information needed by each certification level is pointed out in the margin of the series books. Series titles *Certified Ophthalmic Assistant Exam Review* and *Certified Ophthalmic Technician Exam Review* each contain an appendix to refer CPOA and CPOT exam-takers to questions that pertain to their exams as well, although the older designations of OptA and OptT are used, respectively.

OPHTHALMIC MEDICAL PERSONNEL

Those assisting in ophthalmology, generically known as ophthalmic medical personnel (OMP), can be certified at three levels: certified ophthalmic assistant (COA), certified ophthalmic technician (COT), and certified ophthalmic medical technologist (COMT). Their certifying body is the Joint Commission on Allied Health Personnel in Ophthalmology (JCAHPO), which owns the trademark rights to the certification designations.

Those who wish to take the computer-based examinations in ophthalmology must first qualify. One option is to enroll in a formal training program leading to the desired credential.

Most OMPs, however, are job trained. In this case, you must qualify by working in the field for a specified length of time. Your physician-sponsor must sign a form indicating that you are proficient at certain tasks. You must also hold current CPR credentials. Job-trained COT candidates must hold the COA title, and COMT applicants must already have their COT. At the COA level, one must first take and pass either the American Academy of Ophthalmology (AAO) Independent Study Course or the Canadian Home Study Course. At the COT and COMT levels, increasing amounts of approved continuing education credits are required. In addition, once the candidate has passed the written exam for the COT or COMT, a practical exam must be taken as well. (Contact JCAHPO for up-to-date details.)

The exam at the COA level includes questions covering history taking (presenting complaint/history of presenting illness, past ocular history, family history, systemic illness [past and present], medications, allergies and drug reactions, partially sighted patient), basic skills and lensometry (methods of measuring/recording acuity, color vision testing, lensometry, A-scan biometry, exophthalmometry, Amsler grid, Schirmer's tests, evaluation of pupils, estimation of anterior chamber depth), patient services (ocular dressings and shields, drug delivery, spectacle principles, assisting patients, minor surgery), basic tonometry (indentation, applanation, non-contact, complications/contraindications, scleral rigidity, factors altering intraocular pressure), instrument maintenance (15 different classes of instruments), and general medical knowledge (CPR, anatomy, physiology, systemic diseases, ocular diseases, ocular emergencies, metric conversions, microbial control).

The prospective COT exam covers COA level material as well as clinical optics (optics, retinoscopy, refractometry, advanced spectacle principles, low vision aids), basic ocular motility (EOM actions, strabismus, amblyopia detection, evaluation assessment methods), visual fields (visual pathways, visual fields, methods of measuring the visual field, techniques, errors in testing, defects from disease), contact lenses (basic principles, fitting procedures, patient instruction, trouble-shooting problems, verification of lenses), intermediate tonometry (aqueous humor dynamics, glaucoma), ocular pharmacology (types, strengths, actions, and complications of over 13 drug classes), and photography (basics, fundus photography, defects/artifacts). The skills evaluation (practical exam) includes lensometry, retinoscopy/refinement, detection and identification of phoria or tropia using appropriate cover tests, either automated or nonautomated visual field testing, keratometry, and simulated applanation tonometry.

Candidates for the COMT level are tested on the COA and COT content areas in addition to microbiology (inflammatory response, microscopy, staining, culture media, specimen collection and processing), advanced tonometry (pathophysiology of glaucoma, tonometry theory, managing tonometry problems), advanced visual fields (advanced principles of testing, etiology, and description of less common defects), advanced color vision (physiology/theory, defects, advanced testing techniques), advanced clinical optics (advanced refractometry, advanced optics), advanced ocular motility (amblyopia, anatomy/physiology of EOMs, binocular function, advanced strabismus), advanced photography (fluorescein angiography, slit lamp, external, specular micrography, film processing), advanced pharmacology (basic concepts of topical medications, mechanism of action and desired effects), special instruments and techniques (13 techniques, including lasers), and advanced general medical knowledge (ocular manifestation of systemic diseases, low vision/blindness, ocular disease, and trauma). During the practical exam, they must calibrate, adjust, and perform applanation tonometry; retinoscopy (plus or minus cylinder), cross cylinder, refinement of refractive error; keratometry; lensometry (read power and mark centers of spectacle lenses), frame measurements, lens clock, PD, near point of accommodation (NPA), amplitude of accommodation, vertex distance, measure contact lenses (power, thickness, and base curve); cover test, prism measurement, Maddox rod measurement, and range of motion; near point of convergence (NPC), duction limitations, convergence and divergence, stereo acuity; demonstrate ability to take fundus photos, load and unload film, identify errors in technique of fundus photos, identify phases of fluorescein angiography from photographs.

In order to keep one's credentials (whether obtained through a formal program or independently), proof of continuing education must be submitted periodically. Continuing education credits are given for JCAHPO-approved classes and self-study.

For current exam criteria, contact:
JCAHPO
2025 Woodland Dr.
St. Paul, MN 55125-2995
Phone: 1-888-284-3937 or 651-731-2944
E-mail: jcahapo@jcahpo.org
Website: www.jcahpo.org

For the ophthalmic assisting home study courses, contact:

AAO
Clinical Education Division
P.O. Box 7424
San Francisco, CA 94120
Phone: 415-561-8540
Fax: 415-561-8575
or
Southern Alberta Institute of Technology
1301 16th Ave, NW
Calgary, Alberta, Canada T2M OL4
Phone: 403-284-8456

There is a rich source of printed material to assist a willing learner in achieving higher levels of education. *The Basic Bookshelf for Eyecare Professionals* (a set of 24 books by SLACK Incorporated) offers *Certified Ophthalmic Assistant Exam Review*, *Certified Ophthalmic Technician Exam Review*, and *Certified Ophthalmic Medical Technologist Review*, which provide hundreds of exam-type questions in every content area. These books are useful for exam candidates as well as for general review. JCAHPO has developed a study guide for COA and COT applicants, each including 20 sample questions, available at the address or website listed on p. 306.

Most of the material in this appendix is reprinted and updated with permission from Borover B, Langley T. *Office and Career Management for the Eyecare Paraprofessional.* Thorofare, NJ: SLACK Incorporated; 1997.

Websites
Related to Eyecare

Note: The number of websites pertaining to eyecare is tremendous; it was impossible to list them all, so this is just a select few (especially in the Manufacturers/Suppliers section). In addition, sites periodically change their URLs or cease altogether. (Be warned: sometimes abandoned sites are taken over by other, surprising folks!) We have done our best to ensure that this listing is accurate as of publication time. There are many good sites that are not listed because of space and time constraints; however, most of those given here also have links to other such sites. It is also important to note that while we've separated sites into categories, some sites offer multiple services (eg, have membership information as well as patient education articles).

PROFESSIONAL ORGANIZATIONS

MedMark
www.medmark.org/oph/oph.html
The ultimate link site for organizations (both professional and public) on all things eye related; also institutes, clinics, colleges, education/training, consumer sites, general, information sources, journals, projects, and much more.

American Academy of Ophthalmology (AAO)
www.aao.org
Includes news, official journals, meeting announcements, member search, links, member services, and patient information.

American Academy of Optometry (AAO)
www.aaopt.org
Includes news from AAO, meeting announcements, links, optometry bulletin board, member services, and patient information.

American Association of Certified Orthoptists (AACO)
www.orthoptics.org
Includes training, continuing education, chats, journal, and links.

American Board of Ophthalmology (ABO)
www.abop.org
Includes history and mission statement; examination application, requirements, dates, and deadlines; requirements for recertification; links; and patient information.

American Medical Association (AMA)
www.ama-assn.org
Includes news, publications, patient information, and member services.

American Optometric Association (AOA)
www.aoanet.org
Primarily for the general public (patient information, media information, links to state optometry associations) but also includes member services, news, meeting information, and policy statements.

American Society of Cataract and Refractive Surgery (ASCRS)
www.ascrs.org
Includes news from ASCRS, official journals, member search, meeting announcements, links, member services, and patient information.

American Society of Ophthalmic Plastic and Reconstructive Surgery (ASOPRS)

www.asoprs.org

Includes member directory, fellowships, official journals, meeting announcements, links, member services, information on activities of ASOPRS Foundation, and patient information.

American Society of Ophthalmic Registered Nurses (ASORN)

http://webeye.ophth.uiowa.edu/ASORN

Includes information on educational programs and certification, publications, member services, and job listings.

Association of Technical Personnel in Ophthalmology (ATPO)

www.atpo.org

About ATPO; salary report, newsletter, professional development, membership, links (including formal OMP programs), and online continuing education credits.

Contact Lens Association of Ophthalmologists (CLAO)

www.clao.org

Includes information on membership, publications, and meetings.

International Perimetric Society (IPS)

http://webeye.ophth.uiowa.edu/ips

About perimetry, the IPS, meeting information, IPS news, membership list, IPS proceedings and abstracts, IPS constitution, and perimetry standards.

Joint Commission on Allied Health Personnel in Ophthalmology

www.jcahpo.org

About JCAHPO, ophthalmic medical assisting, certification, education and research foundation, continuing education program listing, news, and events.

Ophthalmic Photographers' Society, Inc

www.opsweb.org

Membership, photo gallery, publications, educational programs, certification, educational information about photography, and informative self-test with explanatory answers.

Opticians Association of America

www.oaa.org

General information, membership information, optician forum, information about continuing education, and website announcements.

Optical Society of America

www.osa.org

Optics and photonics research, applications, and industry news.

Robert B. Scott Ocularists of Florida, Inc

www.ocularist.com

Includes member search, information on publications and meetings, and patient information.

Vitreous Society Online

www.vitreoussociety.org

Vitreous Society online journal, news, annual meeting information, and more.

OTHER ORGANIZATIONS

American Diabetes Association (ADA)
www.diabetes.org
Primarily for patients but also has information for health care professionals. Includes news of interest to diabetics; association news, publications, and services; diabetes research information; and links.

Association for Macular Diseases and the Macula Foundation, Inc
www.macula.org
Site for both patients and professionals. Includes detailed information about the eye and macular degeneration (extensive, excellent graphics), activities of association and foundation, research grants, meetings, and links.

Eye Bank Association of America (EBAA)
www.restoresight.org
Includes news, information for patients, member services, and links.

Foundation Fighting Blindness (FFB)
www.blindness.org
Official site of organization supporting research and treatment of retinal degenerative diseases.

The Glaucoma Foundation
www.glaucoma-foundation.org
Includes information on research programs, donations, patient information, news, and publications.

Lighthouse International Low Vision Resources and Information
www.lighthouse.org/resources_main.htm
Publications, resources, courses, advocacy, eye conditions, eyecare, low vision, newsletters, volunteers, and links.

Low Vision Council
www.lowvisioncouncil.org
The Low Vision Council is an international group of manufacturers, practitioners, educators, agencies, and associations working together to raise awareness of low vision rehabilitation among eyecare providers, as well as visually impaired consumers and their caregivers.

Macular Degeneration Foundation
www.eyesight.org
Patient education and support on macular degeneration and related conditions of low vision.

National Association for Visually Handicapped
www.navh.org
For patients, family, and friends who need everything from large print books to the latest on their particular condition. Health care professionals are welcome here as well. Tips for the visually impaired on reconfiguring web browsers and more.

National Eye Institute
www.nei.nih.gov
News items, funding availability, and links to several full- text pamphlets and booklets for the general public. Topics include age-related macular degeneration, cataract, diabetic retinopathy, and glaucoma.

Prevent Blindness America

www.prevent-blindness.org

National voluntary health agency working to prevent blindness. The site contains eye facts and fun, including eye health and safety tips, glaucoma information, and the effects of computers on your eyes.

REFERENCE (PROFESSIONAL)

Atlas of Ophthalmic Images

www.eyeatlas.com

Color photos of the eye and ocular conditions Includes an invitation to contribute your own photos.

The Eye Exam

www.medicine.ucsd.edu/clinicalmed/eyes.htm

Takes you through a virtual eye exam, including photos of normal and disorders; how to's: external exam, visual acuity, extraocular muscles, visual field, pupil evaluation, and direct ophthalmoscopy.

Eye Lesson

www.yorku.ca/eye/eye1.htm

A simple one-page interactive diagram useful for understanding the basic anatomy of the eye.

eyetec.net

www.eyetec.net

Hints on passing JCAHPO certification exams and online continuing education credits.

Handbook of Ocular Disease Management

www.emedicine.com/oph/index.shtml

Information on how to manage over 50 commonly encountered ocular diseases, signs and symptoms, underlying pathophysiology, recommendations on treatment, and clinical pearls.

Medical Matrix: Ophthalmology
www.medmatrix.org
Peer-reviewed, updated clinical resources for ophthalmology. Register to use, then click on "Ophthalmology" from the index page. Links to organizations, procedures, practice guidelines, searches, news, journals, patient education, directories, cases, educational materials, images, continuing education, classifieds, and forums.

Merck Manual of Diagnosis and Therapy Ophthalmologic Disorders
www.merck.com/pubs/mmanual/section8/sec8.htm
Thirteen chapters on the eye from the 17th edition of the *Merck Manual of Diagnosis and Therapy.*

National Library of Medicine
www.nlm.nih.gov
Health information, library services, research programs, and clinical trials. Health information offers Medlineplus (medical encyclopedia and dictionaries, drug information, current health news, patient education) and Medline/Pub Med (searches 4300 biomedical journals). Also information on AIDS/HIV, cancer, health services, toxicology, and more.

JOURNALS

American Journal of Ophthalmology (AJO)
www.ajo.com
Table of contents, information for contributors, links, and some other information available for free. Most content requires paid subscription.

American Orthoptic Journal (AOJ)

www.aoj.org

Site of the official journal of American Association of Certified Orthoptists (AACO). Includes table of contents, searchable abstracts, continuing medical education quiz, subscription and contributor information, and some information on AACO.

Contact Lens Spectrum

www.clspectrum.com

Includes table of contents, back issues, news, patient information, and subscriptions.

Digital Journal of Ophthalmology (DJO)

www.djo.harvard.edu

Includes online articles, grand rounds, CD-ROM reviews, links, and information for patients and contributors.

Ocular Surgery News

www.osnsupersite.com

A news magazine designed for ocular professionals. Full-text news items, information about conferences and meetings, and full-color discussions of current surgical techniques.

Ophthalmic Journals on the World Wide Web

www.medbioworld.com/med/journals/opth.html

This is the ultimate for finding optometric and ophthalmic journals, with links to nearly 100 professional journals.

Primary Care Optometry News

www.pconsupersite.com

Table of contents, search program, full-text articles, online seminar, special forum, and shopping.

20/20 Magazine
www.2020mag.com
Information on lenses and frames. Features include lab watch, market watch, fashion, continuing education, research; for eyecare professionals and eyewear retailers.

SUPPLIERS/MANUFACTURERS

Akorn
www.akorn.com
Pharmaceutical/medical products; ophthalmic products: surgical instruments and products, pharmaceuticals, and medical office products.

Alcon
www.alconlabs.com
Consumer/professional information; products (over-the-counter: contact lens care, lubricants; prescription: glaucoma, allergy, infection, etc; IOLs, LASIK), conditions, and studies.

Allergan
www.allergan.com
Product information for eyecare professionals and consumers. Products: neurotoxin, contact lens care, surgical products, therapeutics (glaucoma, infection, allergy, etc).

American Optical
www.aolens.com
Custom precision optical products (design, coatings, etc), standard optical products (stock acrylic lenses and molds).

Bausch & Lomb

www.bausch.com

Contact lenses and supplies, patient education on conditions/treatments, pharmaceutical products (glaucoma, vitamins, allergy, etc), microsurgical instruments.

CIBA Vision

www.cibavision.com

Contact lenses and supplies, surgical and IOLs; also patient education on many vision/eye topics.

Johnson & Johnson

www.jnjvision.com

Patient education on contacts; professionals need a company-supplied code to log on to the professional area.

Marco Ophthalmics

www.marcooph.com

Ophthalmic products (refractors, slit lamps, stands, trial sets, projectors, etc), distributors, and conventions.

Medical Ophthalmics

www.medicalophthalmics.com

Vitamins; online and printable brochures on various topics, mostly nutritional.

Novartis Ophthalmics

www.novartisophthalmics.com

Parent company of CIBA; professional and consumer sites; product listing, eye condition information, articles, and media.

OptiSearch

www.optisearch.com

Over 18,000 frames online: search by manufacturer, collection, specifications, or product. Also offers manufacturer directory.

Precision Optical Co
www.precision-optical-co.com
Products (lenses, frames, sunglasses, etc), services (full lab services), and specials.

SOLA Optical
www.sola.com
Patient education on vision and eyeglasses; professional information for labs, retail, and offices; technical articles on lens design, etc.

Zeiss Humphrey Systems
www.humphrey.com
Sales, service, news, and events.

Suggested Reading

American Academy of Ophthalmology. *Pediatric Ophthalmology and Strabismus: Section Six*. San Francisco, Calif: Author; 1993.

American Academy of Ophthalmology. *Optics, Refraction, and Contact Lenses: Section Three* (Basic and Clinical Science Course #0280030). San Francisco, Calif: Author; 2000.

American Optometric Association, AOA Paraoptometric Section. *Self-Study Course for Optometric Assisting*. 2nd ed. Burlington, Mass: Butterworth-Heinemann Medical; 1997.

Anderson DR, Patella VM. *Automated Static Perimetry*. 2nd ed. St. Louis, Mo: Mosby-Year Book; 1999.

Bartlett JD, Jaanus SD. *Clinical Ocular Pharmacology*. 4th ed. Burlington, Mass: Butterworth-Heinemann Medical; 2001.

Bittinger M. *General Medical Knowledge for Eyecare Paraprofessionals*. Thorofare, NJ: SLACK Incorporated; 1999.

Borover B, Langley T. *Office and Career Management for the Eyecare Paraprofessional*. Thorofare, NJ: SLACK Incorporated; 1997.

Boess-Lott R, Stecik S. *The Ophthalmic Surgical Assistant*. Thorofare, NJ: SLACK Incorporated; 1999.

Boyd BF. *LASIK and Beyond LASIK: Wavefront Analysis and Customized Ablation*. Thorofare, NJ: SLACK Incorporated; 2001.

Brady FB. *A Singular View: The Art of Seeing With One Eye*. 5th ed. Annapolis, Md: Author; 1988.

Brown B. *The Low Vision Handbook.* Thorofare, NJ: SLACK Incorporated; 1997.

Budenz DL. *Atlas of Visual Fields.* Philadelphia, Pa: Lippincott, Williams & Wilkins; 1997.

Buratto L. *Corneal Topography: The Clinical Atlas.* Thorofare, NJ: SLACK Incorporated; 1996.

Carlson NB. *Clinical Procedures for Ocular Examination.* 2nd ed. New York, NY: McGraw-Hill Professional Publishing; 1996.

Carlton J. *Frames and Lenses.* Thorofare, NJ: SLACK Incorporated; 2000.

Casser L, Fingeret M, Woodcome HT. *Atlas of Primary Eyecare Procedures.* 2nd ed. New York, NY: McGraw-Hill Professional Publishing; 1997.

Cassin B. *Fundamentals for Ophthalmic Technical Personnel.* Philadelphia, Pa: WB Saunders; 1995.

Chen WYW. *The Pocket Guide to Ophthalmology Review.* Thorofare, NJ: SLACK Incorporated; 2000.

Choplin N, Edwards R. *Visual Fields.* Thorofare, NJ: SLACK Incorporated; 1998.

Choplin NT, Edwards RP. *Visual Field Testing with the Humphrey Field Analyzer: A Text and Clinical Atlas.* 2nd ed. Thorofare, NJ: SLACK Incorporated; 1999.

Contact Lens Association of Ophthalmologists. *Contact Lenses: The CLAO Guide to Basic Science and Clinical Practice.* 2nd ed. New York, NY: Little, Brown & Co; 1989.

Corboy JM. *The Retinoscopy Book: An Introductory Manual for Eye Care Professionals.* 4th ed. Thorofare, NJ: SLACK Incorporated; 1995.

Cunningham D. *Clinical Ocular Photography.* Thorofare, NJ: SLACK Incorporated; 1998.

Daniels K. *Contact Lenses.* Thorofare, NJ: SLACK Incorporated; 1999.

Dickson C. *Low Vision: Principles and Practice.* Burlington, Mass: Butterworth-Heinemann Medical; 1998.

DuBois L. *Basic Procedures.* Thorofare, NJ: SLACK Incorporated; 1998.

Duvall B, Kershner RM. *Ophthalmic Medications and Pharmacology.* Thorofare, NJ: SLACK Incorporated; 1998.

Duvall BS, Lens A, Werner EB. *Cataract and Glaucoma for Eyecare Paraprofessionals.* Thorofare, NJ: SLACK Incorporated; 1999.

Eskridge JB, Amos JF, Bartlett JD. *Clinical Procedures in Optometry.* Philadelphia, Pa: Lippincott, Williams & Wilkins; 1991.

Fannin TE, Grosvenor T. *Clinical Optics.* 2nd ed. Burlington, Mass: Butterworth-Heinemann Medical; 1997.

Fletcher DC, ed. *Low Vision Rehabilitation: Caring for the Whole Person (Ophthalmology Monographs, #12).* San Francisco, Calif: American Academy of Ophthalmology; 1999.

Gayton JL, Kershner RM. *Refractive Surgery for Eyecare Paraprofessionals.* Thorofare, NJ: SLACK Incorporated; 1997.

Gayton JL, Ledford JR. *The Crystal Clear Guide to Sight for Life.* Lancaster, Pa: Starburst Publishers; 1996.

Gimbel HV, Penno AEA. *LASIK Complications: Prevention and Management.* Thorofare, NJ: SLACK Incorporated; 1998.

Goldberg S. *Ophthalmology Made Ridiculously Simple.* 2nd ed. Miami, Fla: Medmaster; 2001.

Gómez Leal A, Muñoz Rodríguez P. *The Atlas of Ophthalmology.* Thorofare, NJ: SLACK Incorporated; 2002.

Gwin N. *Overview of Ocular Disorders.* Thorofare, NJ: SLACK Incorporated; 1999.

Hansen VC. *A Systematic Approach to Strabismus.* Thorofare, NJ: SLACK Incorporated; 1998.

Hargis-Greenshields L, Sims L. *Emergencies in Eyecare.* Thorofare, NJ: SLACK Incorporated; 1999.

Henson DB. *Visual Fields.* Oxford, UK: Oxford University Press; 1996.

Herrin MP. *Instrumentation for Eyecare Paraprofessionals.* Thorofare, NJ: SLACK Incorporated; 1999.

Hunter DG, West CE. *Last Minute Optics: A Concise Review of Optics, Refraction, and Contact Lenses.* Thorofare, NJ: SLACK Incorporated; 1996.

Johnston RL, Cakanac CJ, eds. *Retina, Vitreous, and Choroid: Clinical Procedures.* Burlington, Mass: Butterworth-Heinemann; 1995.

Jose RT, ed. *Understanding Low Vision.* New York, NY: American Foundation for the Blind; 1983.

Kanski JJ. *Clinical Ophthalmology: A Systematic Approach.* 4th ed. Burlington, Mass: Butterworth-Heinemann; 1999.

Kline LB, Bajandas FJ. *Neuro-Ophthalmology Review Manual.* 5th ed. Thorofare, NJ: SLACK Incorporated; 1996.

Kooijman AC, Looijestijn PL, Welling JA, eds. *Low Vision.* Amsterdam, The Netherlands: IOS Press; 1994.

Langerhorst CT. *Automated Perimetry in Glaucoma.* Amsterdam, The Netherlands: Kugler Publications/Ghedini Editore; 1988.

Ledford JK. *Certified Ophthalmic Assistant Exam Review Manual.* Thorofare, NJ: SLACK Incorporated; 1997.

Ledford JK. *Certified Ophthalmic Technician Exam Review Manual.* Thorofare, NJ: SLACK Incorporated; 1997.

Ledford JK. *The Complete Guide to Ocular History Taking.* Thorofare, NJ: SLACK Incorporated; 1999.

Ledford JK. *Certified Ophthalmic Medical Technologist Exam Review Manual*. Thorofare, NJ: SLACK Incorporated; 2000.

Ledford JK, ed. *Handbook of Clinical Ophthalmology for Eyecare Professionals*. Thorofare, NJ: SLACK Incorporated; 2001.

Ledford JK, Pineda R. *The Little Eye Book: A Pupil's Guide to Understanding Ophthalmology*. Thorofare, NJ: SLACK Incorporated; 2002.

Ledford JK, Sanders VN. *The Slit Lamp Primer*. Thorofare, NJ: SLACK Incorporated; 1998.

Lens A. *Optics, Retinoscopy, and Refractometry*. Thorofare, NJ: SLACK Incorporated; 1999.

Lens A. *LASIK for Technicians*. Thorofare, NJ: SLACK Incorporated; 2002.

Lens A, Langley T, Nemeth SC, Shea C. *Ocular Anatomy and Physiology*. Thorofare, NJ: SLACK Incorporated; 1999.

Milder B, Rubin ML, Weinstein GW. *The Fine Art of Prescribing Glasses Without Making a Spectacle of Yourself*. 2nd ed. Gainesville, Fla: Triad Publishing Company; 1991.

Nelson LB. *Pediatric Ophthalmology*. Philadelphia, Pa: WB Saunders; 1984.

Pavan-Langston D, ed. *Manual of Ocular Diagnosis and Therapy*. 4th ed. New York, NY: Little, Brown & Company; 1995.

Physicians' Desk Reference for Ophthalmic Medicines 2001. 29th ed. Montvale, NJ: Medical Economics Company; 2000.

Pickett K. *Overview of Ocular Surgery and Surgical Counseling*. Thorofare, NJ: SLACK Incorporated; 1999.

Rosenthal BP, ed. *Functional Assessment of Low Vision*. St. Louis, Mo: Mosby-Year Book; 1996.

Rubin ML. *Optics for Clinicians.* Gainesville, Fla: Triad Publishing Company; 1993.

Saine PJ, Tyler ME. *Ophthalmic Photography: A Textbook of Fundus Photography, Angiography, and Electronic Imaging.* Burlington, Mass: Butterworth-Heinemann Medical; 1997.

Scheiman M. *Understanding and Managing Vision Deficits: A Guide for Occupational Therapists.* 2nd ed. Thorofare, NJ: SLACK Incorporated; 2002.

Shingleton BJ, Mead MD. *Handbook of Eye Emergencies.* Thorofare, NJ: SLACK Incorporated; 1998.

Simon JW, Calhoun JH, Parks MM. *A Child's Eyes: A Guide to Pediatric Primary Care.* Gainesville, Fla: Triad Publishing Co; 1998.

Stein HA, Cheskes A, Stein RM. *The Excimer: Fundamentals and Clinical Use.* Thorofare, NJ: SLACK Incorporated; 1995.

Stein HA, Freeman MI, Stein RM, Maund LD. *Contact Lenses: Fundamentals and Clinical Use.* Thorofare, NJ: SLACK Incorporated; 1997.

Stein HA, Slatt BJ, Freeman MI, Stein RM. *Fitting Guide for Rigid and Soft Contact Lenses: A Practical Approach.* 4th ed. St. Louis, Mo: Mosby-Year Book; 2002.

Stein HA, Slatt BJ, Stein RM. *The Ophthalmic Assistant: A Guide for Ophthalmic Medical Personnel.* 7th ed. San Diego, Calif: Harcourt Brace; 2000.

Taylor D, ed. *Pediatric Ophthalmology.* 2nd ed. Boston, Mass: Blackwell Science Inc; 1997.

Van Boemel GB. *Special Skills and Techniques.* Thorofare, NJ: SLACK Incorporated; 1999.

Vaughan DG, Asbury T, Riordan-Eva P, eds. *General Ophthalmology.* 15th ed. New York, NY: McGraw-Hill Professional Publishing; 1998.

Walsh TJ, ed. *Visual Fields: Examination and Interpretation (Ophthalmology Monographs, 3).* San Francisco, Calif: American Academy of Ophthalmology; 1991.

Werner EB, Rossi C. *Manual of Visual Fields (Manuals in Ophthalmology).* Philadelphia, Pa: Churchill Livingstone; 1991.